YOUR MAN'S HEALTH

FIONA MARSHALL has written widely on health, psychology and parenting. She is the author of eight books, five of them for Sheldon Press, and also a novel.

Overcoming Common Problems Series

A full list of titles is available from Sheldon Press,
1 Marylebone Road, London NW1 4DU, and on our website at
www.sheldonpress.co.uk

Overcoming Common Problems Series

Overcoming Common Problems Series

Overcoming Common Problems

Your Man's Health

Fiona Marshall

sheldon PRESS

First published in Great Britain in 2002 by
Sheldon Press
1 Marylebone Road
London NW1 4DU

© Fiona Marshall 2002

British Library Cataloging-in-Publication Data

A catalogue record for this book is available from the British Library

ISBN 0–85969–889–0

1 3 5 7 9 10 8 6 4 2

Typeset by Deltatype Limited, Birkenhead, Merseyside
Printed in Great Britain by Biddles Ltd
www.biddles.co.uk

Contents

To all men who would like
to improve their health

Introduction

What is the future of men? Are men the new women? Will men be needed at all? The last few years have seen several major conferences, magazines, articles, TV and radio programmes and web sites, all focused on male health and posing questions like these. Have they come in time to save the race from extinction? What with the global fall in sperm counts, men's appalling health records, and their relatively short life expectancy, it looks as though males are on a rapid downward slope. Add in sperm banks and human cloning, and men look like becoming a superfluous genus. Some see men as taking an increasingly female role in the world, accepting a range of magazines and TV shows aimed at men with contents identical to traditional 'women's stuff', while women increasingly perform all the tasks and jobs traditionally reserved for men. What seemed set in stone just a couple of decades ago – the future of men in society – looks a lot less certain today.

While some of the questions above may be posed more seriously than others, there are very real reasons for the worries about male health. Men have higher mortality rates for all 15 leading causes of death, including lung cancer, heart disease, accidents and suicide. They are three times as likely to commit suicide as are women. Rates of prostate cancer, which kills 9,000 men a year in the UK (four times as many men as cervical cancer will kill women), have doubled in the last 20 years, while rates of male obesity have trebled. There has also been a rise in psychosocial disorders in men, such as alcoholism, addiction, mid-life crisis, depression, suicide and domestic violence. Men have a much shorter life expectancy than women – seven years on average. If he is a black man and she is a white woman the difference is even greater – 14 years.

Why is this? Why are men in such bad shape? Socially, the balance is in their favour. Compared with women, they may earn more money, have less responsibility for childcare, and be more free to take exercise and look after themselves generally. But, as women catch up with work opportunities and equal pay, some experts believe we may see the gaps in health and life expectancy widen even further – unless women also adopt the self-destructive health patterns of men.

The social behaviour of men seems to be largely what militates against their health. Four out of five men do not visit their doctor when they feel unwell. They are not very interested in preventative health. They take more risks, have more accidents, smoke and drink more, and in general live more dangerously than women. They seem to have a prevalent feeling that it is not their place to look after themselves. Largely because of their poor health habits, they die much earlier than they should. It is important not to think entirely in stereotypes and to stress that this does not apply to all men – some men are highly health-conscious and have no trouble talking about their physical or mental health, while some women hate going to the doctor's, dislike showing emotion, and are fatalistic or careless about their overall health. However, the general picture remains – and, as already stated, is causing a great deal of concern.

Just three decades ago, there was very limited research specifically targeted at women's health. It was more or less assumed that women's health needs were the same as men's. In recent years this has changed. There is increasing recognition that men and women have different health and healthcare needs, with major health studies revealing important differences between the two. A well-publicized example in female health is the effect of certain anti-convulsant drugs on the unborn child of pregnant women with epilepsy; for years these drugs were given to women without adequate recognition that they could cause defects in the baby.

Many feel that this new science of 'his and hers' medicine has a long way to go. An American study, for example, called for scientists and doctors to pay more attention to the basic biological differences between men and women. The study added that clinical trials need to test for differences in how the sexes react to diseases and drugs, and that doctors need to take these differences into account when diagnosing, prescribing and advising on preventative care. In other words, it calls for a whole new overall view of medicine and healthcare, and the way in which it is administered. Lately, it is felt in some quarters that men are losing out on healthcare, and that provision is less well-defined than in women's healthcare.

This is changing – indeed, the very emergence of male health as an issue may be one of the reasons why men's health is often thought of in terms of particular subjects such as the prostate, testicular cancer, or impotence. We have not yet quite got round to viewing male health in a holistic way, although this is slowly arriving. Meanwhile, many feel that there is still a gap between male and female health awareness and healthcare.

The gap, at the moment, is still left to women to fill. Women are traditionally the main force behind men's health, and tend to take the initiative not just in caring for their men, but in educating them about health. Forty per cent of men will only attend their family doctor, especially for preventative care, if their partner tells them to (usually part of the healthcare responsibility for the whole family). A MORI poll found that women have a better understanding of the male body than do men, as well as being generally better informed about health than are men.

There are several reasons why you may find yourself becoming actively involved in your partner's health. For purely altruistic reasons, your involvement can have a profound impact on his ability to heal after an illness. Some research has shown that men whose partners are actively involved in their health tend to recover more quickly, especially after surgery.

It is commonly said that men tend to communicate more by behaviour, and women by means of words (again, like all generalizations to do with the sexes, this statement needs a lot of qualifying). If, however, illness can be viewed as a behaviour, then you may be needed to interpret this behaviour – the reasons behind it, what to do about it, not just in terms of treatment but in wider overall lifestyle decisions.

You may also become involved because his health affects your own health and way of life. For example, the partner of a man with erectile dysfunction may lose out on intimacy, self-esteem and trust. If you are informed about impotence, however, you will know that it can be a symptom of a wide variety of underlying disorders including diabetes and heart trouble, and that even impotence by itself is medically treatable in many ways. Infertility likewise stems from a problem with the male partner around 50 per cent of the time; yet you may blame yourself because you 'can't get pregnant'. Often, what may be felt to be a private shame turns out to be a fairly common health disorder.

Again, being involved in a man's health may be good for your health in other ways, too. A partner's poor health habits may pose a danger to others – a by-product of smoking is passive smoking; alcoholism may result in abuse or car accidents; his refusal to attend to his stress level may result in his no longer being able to cope with his job. Taking this further, if he becomes disabled, your quality of life will be profoundly affected too, and social, sporting, travel and retirement activities may be limited. Finally, death has the ultimate impact on the woman, leaving her alone.

This may sound dramatic, but it is a fact of life for many women. However, there are a number of ways in which you can help your men to better health, starting with a better understanding of male health and possible problems. By being well-informed, you can keep your eyes open for signs and symptoms and encourage your partner to have them checked immediately. You can share what you learn with your partner, perhaps encouraging him to read a book like this one, or an article, or passing on the phone number of an information or support organization. Most men suffer alone, yet research has shown that sharing with other men with the same condition has enormous benefit.

You can accompany him to the doctor – women often have better vocabulary and communication skills when it comes to explaining symptoms and asking questions of medical professionals. Taking this further, you can also be better informed about check-ups – both in terms of what is on offer from the doctor, such as regular cholesterol checks, and what you can do yourself, such as how to check for testicular cancer. Again, you can make a family health history as well as history of his individual health which can be invaluable in identifying possible areas which may need extra attention.

On a day-to-day basis, as many women tend to do the shopping and cooking, responsibility for his healthy diet may well be in your hands. You can also motivate him to exercise – even better, join him!

Last but by no means least, it helps to understand the male approach to health with its accompanying feelings of fear and embarrassment. Above all, you may need to tackle the male feeling of being indomitable: the feeling that he can safely get away with it – whether 'it' is an overly hectic lifestyle, drinking and driving, or refusing to check out that persistent pain in his stomach. It is hoped that this book will help you with this, as with all the above points.

This book looks at various conditions and different aspects of preventative health, but, basically, if you can get your man to take three simple steps, you will have made a major impact on his health. These are to take more physical activity, to eat less, especially less saturated fat, and to eat more vegetables and fruit.

Finally, educating him about his health can also extend to sons. If the next generation's men are to be healthy, now is the time to be starting the process. Once again, women can be enormously influential in changing a culture in which it used to be accepted that men are not really expected to be responsible for their health. While 'fitness' is still a leading definition of health among men (often the only definition), health in its wider aspects, including preventative and emotional, is finally finding a place in what used to be a macho-bound society. Let us hope that the species will survive after all.

Acknowledgements

I am indebted to many who have worked to raise awareness of men's health; in particular, Dr Sarah Brewer, Dr Ian Banks, the Men's Health Forum and CancerBACUP. Thanks also to counsellor Denise Knowles for her sensitive insights.

1

The cardiac factor

Coronary heart disease (CHD) remains the biggest preventative care problem in the western world for the medical profession. The most common cause of death in the UK, it is a leading premature killer of men, accounting for one in four deaths in men, compared with one in six women – as with other aspects of male health, men come off worse than women.

While the number of people dying from heart disease has fallen by 10 per cent in recent years, the number of people actually suffering from coronary heart conditions (around 2.6 million in the UK) has in fact gone up. Lowered death rates are believed to be due to more sophisticated treatment, and the fact that more people are giving up smoking and making changes in their diet. Even so, CHD is still the single biggest killer in the UK, claiming nearly 125,000 lives a year. The death rate from heart and circulatory disease in the UK is still very high compared with other countries – almost twice that of France and well above the European Union average, and also high compared with America or Australia.

Yet, much of the risk can be prevented. Medical experts warn that we need to take action to combat two major lifestyle issues which threaten our health:

- lack of physical activity – around 20 per cent of us do no physical activity at all, while one in three take less than 30 minutes' exercise per week
- obesity – which has trebled in men since the 1980s.

Research shows that the first of these is vital when it comes to preventing CHD. While a healthy diet certainly promotes a healthier weight and heart, exercise has a terrific influence on reducing the risk of heart disease. According to the British Heart Foundation, if the UK's sedentary population (37 per cent of adults) were to do 30 minutes of physical activity five times a week, coronary heart disease deaths could be reduced by around 10 per cent – obviously,

1

increased physical activity also combats obesity. (Today's lifestyle also has implications for our children, who suffer increasingly from obesity and lack of physical activity.) As stated in the Introduction, male health does not exist in a vacuum – his health affects yours and your children's, even if it is only by example.

Is he at risk?

In CHD, the arteries, which supply blood to the heart, become clogged with plaque made up of calcium and cholesterol, causing blood clots to form, a process known as atherosclerosis. As a result, less blood reaches the heart, and so less oxygen, causing muscle cramping and pain (the latter known as angina). If the process continues and worsens, muscle cells become damaged and die. The most common forms of CHD are angina and heart attack.

Apart from lack of physical activity and obesity, a number of risk factors for CHD have been identified. Some of these you cannot change – for example, being male in itself poses a higher risk of CHD, as women are protected by oestrogen before menopause. Likewise, the older you are, the more at risk you are from CHD. For many factors, however, it is possible to do something. Risk factors include:

- smoking – 20 cigarettes a day doubles the risk of CHD. A WHO (World Health Organization) report showed that half of all smokers will die as a direct result of cigarettes. Smoking makes the blood more prone to clotting and so can lead to atherosclerosis. It also reduces available oxygen and destroys vitamin C, which protects the heart. Smoking in combination with other risk factors makes heart disease even more likely; for example, high blood pressure and smoking together damage blood vessels more quickly than either alone;
- uncontrolled high blood pressure – see below;
- high cholesterol levels (of LDL cholesterol) – see below;
- poorly controlled diabetes;
- too much alcohol;
- a diet high in saturated fats, cholesterol and sugar;
- area – some areas, such as Scotland, have a higher rate of CHD;
- lower social class;

2

- family history – having a family history of premature (under 60 years) CHD.

Stress, personality and the heart

Stress and how we respond to it can affect the heart and circulation, as prolonged stress may raise blood pressure to levels which can put him more at risk. So major life events such as bereavement, job loss, illness, or divorce can increase the risk depending on how he reacts to them.

Certain types of personality have also been associated with a greater risk of heart trouble, classically the so-called Type A personality, said to be aggressive, driven and success-orientated. Recent research has refined this concept, showing that having 'Type A' qualities do not themselves put men at greater risk of a heart attack. The key factor seems to be how angry he gets. Several studies have shown that men who have an angry approach to life and who easily become angry have a four to five times greater risk of developing heart disease at an early age compared with men who are calmer.

The 'flight or fight' response we have when under intense stress means that the heart rate increases because of the increased adrenaline. Blood vessels dilate to allow blood to travel faster to your muscles, while the blood thickens to lessen any bleeding that would occur if you were to be injured. Persistent repetition of this kind of response is a major stress on the heart and arteries and may lead to damage.

Anger can even lessen the amount of oxygen a man's heart receives during exercise – over a sustained period of time, this can lead to heart disease as the heart becomes increasingly starved of oxygen. On the positive side, exercise is a great way of releasing this anger.

Stress has an inherent physiological component – it is not all personality. For example, black men are at far greater risk of high blood pressure than are white men, and nearly twice as many die of strokes. Some American research which looked at

3

how people respond to stress found that the blood vessels of males and females, and of blacks and whites, reacted quite differently. The blood vessels of white women constricted less under stress than did those of white men, and black men showed greater constriction than either group. The greater the constriction, the higher the blood pressure. This study highlights how important it is for men, especially black men, to do their best to reduce the stress in their lives.

For suggestions on how to deal with stress, see Chapter 9.

Angina

Angina, or angina pectoris, affects five out of every thousand men in the UK over the age of 40 and can occur by itself, or be the precursor of a heart attack. Angina is chest pain caused by the narrowing of the arteries as they become furred up with a fatty substance called atheroma.

Symptoms include severe pain in the chest, radiating to the neck and left arm, a tight feeling in the chest and sometimes pain between the shoulder blades. The pain most usually happens after physical exertion, a heavy meal, cold weather, emotional stress, or any other circumstances which may cause the heart to work harder than usual.

As the arteries become more blocked, pain comes on with less exertion, or even at rest, and takes longer to ease off. Known as crescendo or unstable angina, this needs urgent treatment to prevent the coronary arteries becoming completely blocked.

Heart attack

Heart attack, or coronary thrombosis or myocardial infarction (MI), is the leading cause of death in men in the UK. An attack, which can strike without warning, happens when the blood supply to the heart is blocked, preventing the passage of essential oxygen and nutrients. As a result, part of the heart muscle dies.

Symptoms include severe, crushing pain across the centre of the chest, which persists for at least 20 minutes. The pain spreads into the neck, jaw, shoulders and arms, accompanied by sweating, nausea, vomiting, palpitations, dizziness and breathlessness.

Urgent treatment is essential as the first few minutes are the most important and, after that, the first three or four hours. If a heart attack is suspected, call an ambulance, have an aspirin (this reduces further blood clotting), and rest until the ambulance arrives.

Heart attacks are not necessarily fatal, but they do leave the heart in a weaker state and not as strong at pumping blood around the body.

Heart failure

Heart failure does not mean that the heart stops. This term is used to describe the condition when the heart cannot produce enough blood to meet the body's demands for oxygen and nutrients. It may be the result of different forms of heart disease. Depending on whether the right or left side of the heart is affected, symptoms include breathlessness, blueness of the skin (cyanosis), and the accumulation of fluid, especially around the ankles (oedema).

Stroke

Men are more likely to suffer a stroke than women – four times more likely, one American study showed. Most victims are over 50, although it can happen at any age. Stroke happens when a blood clot deprives part of the brain of oxygen. Full stroke includes this and loss of bowel control and consciousness, and difficulty swallowing.

Minor strokes, known as TIAs (transient ischaemic attacks), may herald a bigger one. Symptoms include slight pins and needles in the arm, leg and side of the face, problems with speech and sight, including brief loss of either or both.

Palpitations

The average heart beats around 72 times a minute and pumps around 5 litres of blood a minute; during exercise the pumping action increases three- or fourfold in response to the extra demand for oxygen.

Palpitations, fast or irregular heartbeats, are common and usually harmless, although they can be frightening. They may occur after exercise, or as a result of too much caffeine or nicotine, or after a shock. They can however be a symptom of heart disease, especially if accompanied by dizziness, faintness, or chest pain, so if they occur frequently it is worth getting them checked by your GP.

High cholesterol and heart disease

High levels of cholesterol are the main cause of the plaque which furs up the arteries, so literally paving the way for heart disease. It is quite possible to have high cholesterol without suspecting it and it is extremely common, affecting a staggering seven out of 10 men.

Cholesterol itself is a fat which the body needs for several functions, such as keeping cells and nerves healthy. There are two types:

- LDL – low density LDL cholesterol, which is the harmful or 'bad' type as its molecules are small enough to pass into the artery walls and clog them (atherosclerosis).
- HDL – high density HDL cholesterol, which is the 'good' type as it is too large to pass into the artery walls and so stays in the bloodstream to carry fats round the body and neutralize the harmful effects of LDL.

Your male partner should have his cholesterol level checked every two years after the age of 30. This is more important if he smokes, is overweight, has high blood pressure, diabetes, a family history of chest pains or heart trouble. A check-up is also a good idea if he has obvious facial signs of high cholesterol, such as yellow deposits around the eyes or a white ring around the iris.

If his cholesterol level is higher than it should be, adjusting what he eats is the first step in getting it down, particularly reducing saturated fats (see below under 'What you can do', and Chapter 6, for diet suggestions). Bear in mind that diet is only one risk factor for CHD, so do not become too obsessed with this.

Your GP may suggest medication to lower his cholesterol, although not everyone feels happy with this.

Iain's GP wanted to put him on pills right away for high cholesterol but Iain asked for three months' grace to try dietary measures first. During this time he cut out red meat and fried foods, while eating more fruit and vegetables. Breakfast was oatmeal with chopped apple, both known to help keep cholesterol

6

levels healthy. Lunch might be yellow pea soup (pulses again are good for cholesterol levels) and dinner, oily fish, salad and baked potatoes. He also started a rigorous exercise programme, training three times a week at the local gym. When he returned to his doctor he had lost a stone in weight and his cholesterol levels had dropped enough for him to avoid medication.

If your partner does have a cholesterol check, he can ask how much of raised levels are in the form of HDL and how much as LDL – if the former, this offers protection from heart disease.

High blood pressure and heart disease

Blood pressure is the force with which the circulating blood presses against the walls of your arteries. In high blood pressure, or hypertension, this force is greater than normal and eventually causes narrowing and thickening of the arteries, so putting extra strain on the heart.

In the USA at least 50 million people have hypertension, while it is also very common in the UK, affecting 10 to 20 per cent. In young adulthood and early middle age it is more common in men than in women; afterwards, more common in women. Obesity and a high intake of sugar and alcohol make you more prone to high blood pressure. Ethnic origin is another factor – for example, hypertension is most prevalent in Japan and northern China, and more common in African Americans than in white Americans. In societies which use little or no salt, hypertension is much lower. Your family history also plays a part as do diabetes, kidney disease and pregnancy.

In mild hypertension there are no symptoms but severe hypertension includes headaches, shortness of breath, visual disturbances and giddiness. Severe hypertension can lead to complications such as damage to parts of the body such as the heart, kidneys or eyes, so it is important to have your blood pressure checked regularly.

What you can do

As already stated, there are a number of ways in which you can help him cut the risk of CHD quite dramatically. It really is a case of small changes making a big difference. If everyone reduced their salt

7

intake as outlined below, for example, the risk of stroke would be cut by a quarter, and the risk of CHD cut by 15 per cent.

However, research has shown that it is more effective to think in terms of an overall healthy lifestyle, rather than just changing one factor like diet. People who combine, say, exercise and diet changes along with stress management and meditation have seen their heart health improve greatly. Likewise, having two or more risk factors together – for example, being very stressed and eating a high-fat, salty diet – make heart disease more likely. The more comprehensive your action plan, the better.

This is even more important if your partner has a close relative who has or has had CHD, in which case you might suggest he takes extra care and perhaps has a talk with his doctor.

John's father died of a heart attack after putting on a lot of weight – he had also been a heavy smoker. Partly because of this, John took a job which ensured he would have a lot of physical activity (he trained as a PE teacher), and never started smoking. One of John's friends at the school, Phil, also had heart disease in the family but believed that red wine was the best preventative – rather too much so, according to his wife Sue! She and John persuaded Phil to limit his alcohol intake and help with a school football club on Saturday mornings so that he got more exercise. Sue also suggested that Phil walk the mile to the school instead of drive.

How to help him

- First and foremost, convince him that he must give up smoking. See the section on giving up smoking in Chapter 9, 'Other lifestyle factors'.
- Encourage him to lose weight if he needs to, or join him in a healthy eating and exercise plan – men who are overweight are one and a half times more likely to have a heart attack than those of healthy weight. If either of you have not exercised for a while, or are very overweight, check first with your GP. If nothing else, get some brisk walking three times a week for about 20 to 30 minutes.
- Encourage him to improve his diet in general. In particular, avoid saturated fat such as fry-ups, fish and chips, fatty meat; full-fat

8

milk, cream, full-fat cheese and butter; cakes, pastries, savoury snacks and biscuits. Grill, roast, boil or steam instead of fry.

- Salt is one of the easier substances to cut down on, so make the most of it and avoid salt as far as possible, not just obviously salty foods such as olives and salami, but foods which contain hidden salt such as processed food, tinned food including soups and vegetables, sauces, stock cubes and preparations, and biscuits. Replace salt with spices, and allow a couple of weeks to retrain your taste buds.

- Eat oily fish such as sardines, herring, salmon and mackerel as they contain omega-3 fats which reduce the blood's tendency to clot, lower levels of cholesterol, lower blood pressure, and reduce the furring up of arteries which causes heart disease.

- Eat more whole foods which contain fibre – oatmeal, apples, beans, peas and pulses may all help keep cholesterol levels healthy if eaten regularly.

- Vitamin E helps fight free radicals which can pave the way to heart disease. Consider taking a supplement or eat foods rich in vitamin E such as wheatgerm, soybeans, vegetable oils, broccoli, leafy green vegetables, whole grains, peanuts, eggs (but bear in mind that eggs are high in cholesterol – UK heart associations recommend two to four eggs a week for the general population).

- Some research shows that sunlight can lower blood pressure, make the heart more efficient, reduce levels of cholesterol, as well as helping weight loss and increasing the level of sex hormones. Not only does sunlight produce vitamin D on the skin, vital for several body functions, it also encourages physical activity – it is much easier to go for a walk on a nice sunny day than on an overcast one. So, encourage him to get more sunlight or at least more daylight, taking common sense measures to protect from sunburn such as avoiding the sun during the hottest part of the day from 11 a.m. to 2 p.m. (see Chapter 2 for more on sunlight therapy).

- Eats lots of food rich in vitamin C including citrus fruits, broccoli, other fresh fruit and vegetables (including potatoes!), rosehips and blackcurrants.

- Red wine, famed for its healthy heart properties, contains antioxidants which also help keep blood healthy; however, red grape juice has the same effect – in fact the beneficial effect may last longer without alcohol, according to some research.

- Olive oil and rapeseed oil contain vitamin E and the monounsaturated fat oleic acid which helps lower LDL cholesterol, so use in moderation, especially if he needs to lose weight (one tablespoon of olive oil contains 100 calories).
- Some 'functional foods' are especially designed to lower cholesterol. Foods containing plant sterol ester and plant stanol ester, such as spreads and salad dressings, use substances (phytosterols) found naturally in minute amounts in fruits, vegetables, nuts, seeds, cereals and legumes. An average portion of the spread (around 20g a day) has been shown to lower cholesterol from 8 to 13 per cent. They should be eaten as part of a healthy diet containing lots of fresh fruit and vegetables.
- Identify sources of stress and help him plan to change them. Among its other benefits, exercise is about the most effective way there is of dealing with stress – even brisk walking. Stress aids may also help, such as traditional herbal remedies and self-help cassettes.
- Help him plan ways of relaxing, for example by researching a new hobby.
- He should get his blood pressure checked at least every five years, and once a year if he is over 55.
- He should also have his cholesterol level checked (see above).
- His GP can also test the urine for diabetes.
- If he seems to be at risk, for example, with a strong family history of heart disease, he could consider taking half an aspirin a day (150mg) to help prevent blood clotting. He should discuss this first with his GP.
- Encourage him to think positively. Men who laugh and think positively are less likely to have a heart attack than men with more negative attitudes.

Nutrients, herbs and oils

While many of the suggestions below are dietary, and can easily be incorporated into a healthy eating plan, he should consult his doctor before undertaking alternative or complementary remedies for heart trouble. In particular, he should not take herbal remedies while taking medication without consulting his doctor.

- Garlic has been shown to lower blood pressure and cholesterol levels, so eat it as raw as you can, i.e. in garlic mayonnaise, or cooked in stews and sauces, or take garlic tablets.
- Hawthorn berries infused in boiling water for 10 minutes are a traditional home remedy to strengthen the heart, lower blood pressure and relax arteries.
- Regular infusions of limeflowers are said to act as tonics for the heart and circulation.
- Rosemary, fresh, dried or as an oil, can be used to boost the circulation.
- Lavender oil can be used in the bath, in a vaporizer or as a gentle massage to help regulate the heart.
- To improve artery health, eat foods rich in bioflavonoids which protect the capillaries and prevent them from bleeding. Good sources include the white pithy core of citrus fruits; also, citrus fruits, apricots, cherries, green peppers and broccoli.
- For high blood pressure, increase your intake of potassium, calcium and magnesium which help balance circulation and encourage heart action. It is better to eat these in foods, rather than as supplements, as too much potassium can cause problems. Sources of potassium include fresh fruit and vegetables, especially bananas, dried apricots, pulses, mushrooms, potatoes and spinach. Sources of magnesium include brown rice, soybeans, nuts, brewer's yeast, whole wheat flour and legumes. Foods rich in calcium include milk, cheese and other dairy products; leafy green vegetables; hard tap water or bottled mineral water with high calcium content; salmon; tinned fish; eggs; beans, including baked beans; nuts; sesame seeds; and tofu.

When to see the doctor

It is worth getting your partner to attend the doctor's surgery for any of the preventative checks described above – blood pressure, cholesterol and diabetes. If he has been experiencing chest pain or discomfort, especially if it matches the description given in 'Heart attack' (above), he should see his GP or attend Casualty without delay. However, you may not get an instant diagnosis as heart pain can be confused with other conditions such as indigestion or even chest muscle strain, so that tests may be needed to clarify exactly what it is. Your doctor can check your heart rate and perform an ECG (electrocardiogram), a recording of the heart's electrical activity which may show changes and irregularities. However, further tests may be needed as a normal ECG is not an infallible sign that all is well.

Finally, it is also worth getting your man to see the doctor if he – or you – is anxious. Anxiety is by no means to be underrated as a source of distress, and can also contribute to future ill-health. Reassurance that all is well can be of immense value in allowing you both to lead normal, healthy lives.

2
Cancers

Cancer runs a close second to heart disease as a killer disease and shows no sign of releasing its hold. The incidence of cancer in men has risen by more than a third, a rise which is believed to be linked to increasing amounts of environmental pollution. One in three people will get cancer at some time in their lives, and one in four will die from the disease.

Of the 240,000-plus new cases of cancer each year, just over half affect men. According to the government's Office of National Statistics, the three most common cancers for men are lung cancer, prostate cancer and bowel cancer. Three cancers affect only men – prostate, testicular and penile cancers.

Cancer treatment is much more sophisticated than it used to be, and cancer organizations have worked hard to put out the message that a diagnosis of cancer is no longer a death sentence. Even better, much can be done in terms of lifestyle to prevent it happening in the first place. This is especially true of lung cancer, where the preventative measures can be summed up in two words: Don't smoke.

This chapter covers the cancers which pose the greatest risk to men, with prostate cancer being covered in the next chapter.

What is cancer?

The term 'cancer' covers a multitude of conditions but, basically, is used to describe an abnormal development of cells in the body. Normally, new cells only grow in place of those which have died but, in cancer, the cell keeps on dividing and grows into a cluster of cells, or tumours. This tumour may be benign, spreading no further; or malignant, spreading further into the body. Benign tumours are not cancers; malignant ones are. These cancerous tumours are known as carcinomas or sarcomas, depending on whereabouts they are in the body.

13

As cancers are various, so are causes – with the exception of smoking, which is the biggest single cause of cancer. Most cancers are probably caused by a combination of an inherited sensitivity to the condition plus some environmental trigger. Around one in three people who develop cancer have a family history of cancer, and cancers that appear to run most often in families include bowel (25 per cent of cases are hereditary), testicular, prostate, skin and breast cancers. The risk of cancer also increases as you become older. While smoking is the single biggest cause of cancer, other major causes include:

- too much alcohol
- poor diet
- being overweight
- chemicals and environmental pollutions.

Obviously, the more lifestyle factors that are combined, the greater the chances of getting cancer, especially if there is already a genetic predisposition to the disease.

Joe worked in a heavy industrial plant where he was exposed to toxins for 20 years. He took little or no exercise (his job was to drive a pick-up truck round the site); smoked heavily, and ate a poor diet, refusing vegetables because he disliked them. His first wife died of stomach cancer. When he remarried seven years later, his second wife did what she could to introduce a healthier lifestyle, making Joe go for walks and so on, but he remained obstinate about diet and smoking, and it was anyway too late. Though, typically, Joe would not consult a doctor, he suffered pain and a range of other symptoms for around a year before eventually being diagnosed with stomach cancer, his case being so grave that the consultant himself visited their home one Sunday evening to break the news. Sadly, Joe died within six months.

Be alert for symptoms

Different cancers have specific symptoms but, generally, you should be alert for any of the following:

- weight loss
- loss of appetite
- difficulty swallowing
- a sore that will not heal within three to four weeks
- persistent or new cough or hoarseness, especially if coughing up blood
- any change in a mole, wart or coloured skin spot such as bleeding, or changing shape or colour
- changes in bowel or bladder habits such as blackening of stools, blood in stools, severe constipation
- persistent or recurring pain anywhere in the body
- indigestion coming on for the first time in later life
- any unusual growths or lumps.

Any of the above should take your man to the doctor without delay. The quicker any cancer is investigated, the better the prognosis for treatment.

Treatment

Cancer treatment has become much more sophisticated, with much better survival rates than in years gone by. Testicular cancer has a cure rate of more than 90 per cent, while a third of all people with cancer survive for more than five years. Genetic research into cancer means the survival odds may improve even further – and, better still, if men start taking more care of themselves, they may not even become statistics.

There are several treatments for cancer which offer increased hope for survival. New, highly developed drugs, which may obviate the need for surgery, may cause side effects but have the ability to attack cancer cells wherever they are in the body, even if the spread has not been detected. Radiation treatment has also been revolutionized, and is much more precisely targeted at the tumour, so reducing the risk of damage to normal cells. Hormone therapy may be used in hormone-sensitive cancers, including prostate cancer. These treatments may be used alone or may follow some form of surgery, which is usually the initial stage in a range of treatments.

Lung cancer

The good news is that fewer men smoke than before, and there are four times as many non-smokers as smokers. Unfortunately, however, lung cancer is the leading cause of death in men who die from cancer, killing around 100 people a day in the UK. One in 12 men will develop lung cancer, of which there are around 25,500 new cases a year.

Half of all heavy smokers will never reach 70, while even light smokers only have a 60 per cent chance of living until 70. Nearly all lung cancer is due to smoking. The more cigarettes he smokes, and the younger the age at which he started smoking, the bigger the risk of lung cancer. Smoking also causes a third of all cancers.

Warning signs of lung cancer include persistent cough, coughing up blood, and increased shortness of breath. While early treatment can work, less than 8 per cent of men survive for more than five years after diagnosis. Prevention is much better than cure.

Skin cancer

Skin cancer is the second most common cancer in men after lung cancer and also is preventable. More men than women get cancer of the skin, mainly squamous or basal cell carcinomas which are very treatable.

Malignant melanoma is on the increase but it is not certain why. It has been linked with exposure to strong sun, but melanoma is also increasing in the UK, not noted for burning sun. Depletion of the ozone layer has been linked with melanoma as a possible cause, but this area needs more research. Bursts of strong sun on unprotected skin have been linked with skin cancer, and some men are more at risk, for example if they have a job which involves more outdoor work and exposure to sunlight, such as a farm worker or postman. Men with a fair complexion, or one that burns easily in sun, are also more prone to skin cancer, as are those with numerous moles, especially if the moles are large or irregular in shape or colour. Having a close relative who has had skin cancer also warrants paying more attention to preventative care.

Warning signs include any mole which changes shape or colour or starts to bleed, a persistent lump on the lower lip, forehead or tip of ear could be a squamous or basal cell carcinoma.

Natural light and cancer

While there is concern about the links between strong sunlight and skin cancer, some research suggests that more natural light – in moderation – reduces the risk of internal cancers (though too much is still linked with external skin cancers). One American study of prostate cancer showed that mortality declines with increasing sunlight intensity. Studies in the USA and the former USSR have shown similar results with colon and breast cancer.

Vitamin D is thought to be the responsible agent in this. A hormone made (synthesized) in the skin by ultraviolet light, it is known to help prevent the growth of tumours and sunlight is the main source of vitamin D, although it exists in some foods. We are getting increasingly less daylight as we spend more and more time inside or in cars, and there is a lot of speculation that light deprivation leads not just to depression but maybe to other maladies as well (see *Coping with SAD*, Fiona Marshall, Sheldon Press 2002).

Some researchers speculate that many people may be marginally deficient in vitamin D, as vitamin D obtained from food is negligible. This is particularly true of older people, as the body's ability to synthesize vitamin D declines with age. Again, more sun has been shown to lower cholesterol and improve heart function, and this may be because vitamin D helps control the amount of calcium in the blood. While 99 per cent of calcium goes to make the skeleton, the remaining 1 per cent is vital for muscle function, including the heart, and for blood clotting, nerve function, and for the activity of several enzymes. Lack of calcium is nearly always due to vitamin D deficiency.

So, while you do not want him to get sunburn or develop

skin cancer, maybe he could benefit from more regular, moderate exposure to daylight – rather than staying indoors for most of the year and then sunbathing all day long on holiday. He can also remove any glasses (normal spectacles or sunglasses) for at least 20–30 minutes at a time as some research suggests that these prevent some health benefits by blocking the sun's access to the eyes. Do not ignore common sense safety precautions. He should:

- never look directly at the sun
- avoid exposing his skin to strong sunlight, especially between the hours of 11 a.m. and 3 p.m.
- use a high factor sunblock (minimum factor 15) in strong sunlight
- wear a hat with a wide brim
- wear a longsleeved T-shirt or shirt.

You can check his skin regularly, not forgetting his back, paying particular attention to any moles which change in any way – get them checked by your doctor.

Bowel cancer

Cancer of the bowel, or colorectal cancer, is the third most common cancer in men after lung and skin cancer, affecting one in 18 men, with around 16,500 new cases a year. It proves fatal to more men than women, especially after their mid-fifties, but like lung cancer it is preventable to a certain extent, and very treatable in the early stages.

Risk factors include a diet high in meat and fat and low in fibre and fresh fruit and vegetables; a previous history of ulcerative colitis (an inflammatory bowel disorder); having bowel cancer in the family; or a relatively rare disorder polyposis coli which causes growths on the inner lining of the bowel.

Warning signs include diarrhoea or constipation lasting for more than two weeks or any other change in bowel habit, blood or heavy mucus in stools, and a feeling of still wanting to go to the loo after opening the bowels.

Testicular cancer

Although quite rare, only 1 per cent of all cancers in men, with around 1,400 new cases a year, this is the single biggest cancer-related cause of death in young men (between 18–35). The good news is that there has been a 75 per cent fall in the death rate from testicular cancer and, if diagnosed early, it has a cure rate of 96 per cent. Even when the cancer has spread, up to 80 per cent of men can still be cured. However, more than 50 per cent of men consult their doctor after the disease has spread. Once again, early diagnosis is life-saving, but missed out on by men who may be too embarrassed or afraid to go to the doctor.

Cases of testicular cancer have doubled over the last 20 years. Although it isn't known exactly why, certain risk factors have been implicated. Men whose testes failed to descend normally are 36 times more likely to develop this form of cancer than men born with both testicles in the scrotum. Testicular cancer also tends to run in families, so that if your partner has a brother who has had this cancer, his chances are 10 times greater of getting it too. Race also seems to play a part – some evidence shows that white men have a six times greater incidence of testicular cancer than do black men.

Oestrogen in milk has been identified as another factor (not just in testicular cancer, but also in male sterility and cancer of the prostate as well as in birth defects). Substances (phthalates) in plastic food wrappings are also believed to have an oestrogen-like effect. However, this research remains speculative.

Checking the testes

Cancer of the testes, like other cancers, can be quite painless so it is important to examine them regularly.

- Do this while in a bath or shower as the warm water makes the scrotum softer and so easier to feel the testes inside.
- Holding the scrotum lightly in your hand, feel the difference between the testes. It is quite normal for one to be larger and lying lower.

- Gently roll each between thumb and forefinger, and using both hands check for any lumps or swellings. The duct carrying sperm to the penis, the epidermis, is naturally lumpy (along the top and back of the testes).
- Check for any small lumps, hardness, swelling, or tenderness.
- Also check for a feeling of heaviness in the scrotum, or a dull ache in the lower abdomen or groin.

Cancer of the penis

Penile cancer is very rare – there is just one case for every 100,000 men each year in the UK – but uncircumcised men over 60 are at greater risk. The exact cause of penile cancer is unknown, but it is thought to be related to general hygiene. A build-up of smegma under the foreskin is believed to be a factor because it can lead to chronic inflammation. Some skin conditions can also develop into cancer if left untreated.

Good hygiene is the best preventative measure. The penis should be thoroughly washed every day, cleaning behind the foreskin. He should also have any skin inflammation checked, even if it seems relatively minor.

Early diagnosis and treatment lead to a cure rate of more than 95 per cent. However, these are important because cancer of the penis often spreads to other parts of the body in the early stages of the disease.

Warning signs include a small lump on the penis, which may look like a wart or spot and may be painful or painless; a painless sore on the penis; pain and bleeding.

Male breast cancer

This rare cancer is most common in men over 60, and is more common if breast cancer (in men and women) runs in the family. A strong family history of ovarian or colon cancer may also increase the risk.

Very rarely, men with high levels of oestrogen, or those who have been exposed to repeated radiation, may be at increased risk; as are men with a rare genetic syndrome, Klinefelter's syndrome, when a man is born with an extra female chromosome.

Warning signs include the presence of a lump in the breast (the most common symptom), but you should also look out for changes in the size or shape of the breast, ulcers or sores on the skin, or changes to the nipple such as turning in, a discharge or a rash.

Helping him prevent cancer

While no one action is guaranteed to prevent cancer, there is much you can do to reduce his risk. Lifestyle remains an important factor as with all male health.

Pat, 61, a builder, was vastly overweight. He worked hard, starting early and never taking lunch, but would make up for it afterwards with a large dinner and evenings in the pub. He developed bowel cancer, for which he was successfully treated, and completely changed his lifestyle, retiring to Spain. In a year he was back in the UK, saying he was bored! He restarted his building company but delegated most of the work to his team and only took the jobs that appealed to him. He continued to use Spain 'as a health camp' as he put it, cut down his drinking to a moderate pint or so when out, and watched what he ate, though he was less disciplined about this and remained somewhat over-weight.

As Pat's story shows, even moderate changes in lifestyle are better than nothing, but obviously the more you can do to help him look after his health, the better your man's chances of preventing cancer.

- Smoking causes most lung cancer and is responsible for a third of all cancer deaths. Giving up smoking should be an absolute priority. If you smoke, now is an excellent chance for you to break the habit too. He can ask his GP or pharmacist about smoking cessation aids or contact one of the support organiza-tions listed at the end of this book (see 'Useful addresses'). See

also the section on giving up smoking in Chapter 9, 'Other lifestyle factors'.

- Some cancers, such as those of the mouth, tongue, oesophagus, throat and liver, are linked to too much alcohol, so get him to drink sensibly. (See Chapter 9, 'Other lifestyle factors'.)
- Help him lose excess weight. Being overweight increases the risk of cancer by a third. (See Chapter 4, 'Fitness', and Chapter 5, 'The inner man', which deals with obesity.)
- Encourage him to take more physical activity – see Chapter 4, 'Fitness'.
- Educate him to avoid environmental pollution such as car fumes, asbestos, chemicals such as pesticides and fungicides, and other people's cigarette smoke.
- He could consider complementary therapies to help him relax and boost his general well-being, such as aromatherapy, massage, reflexology and acupuncture.

Diet and preventing cancer

Around 25 per cent of cancers in the UK are related to diet, and particular risk factors include eating too much fat (particularly saturated fat), too little fibre and not enough fruit and vegetables containing the vitamins A, C and E. These antioxidant vitamins help wipe out free radicals, which can damage the body's cells and pave the way for cancer. While you should not view diet as a cure for cancer and should be wary of people who claim that a certain diet will banish cancer, you have a better chance of preventing cancer if you make his diet as healthy as possible. Golden rules include:

- Make your diet low-fat – no more than 30 per cent of his calorie intake should come from fat.
- Avoid saturated (animal) fat.
- Eat high-fibre foods (cereals, fruits and vegetables) and plenty of the antioxidant vitamins A, C and E. In particular, plenty of fruit and raw or lightly cooked vegetables are thought to reduce the risk of bowel cancer and WHO

recommends a minimum daily intake of half a kilo of these a day. Eat at least five portions of fruit and vegetables a day. Vegetarians run half the risk of cancer of meat-eaters.

- Increase intake of wholegrain cereals and pulses.
- Reduce salt intake, including foods that have been cured, pickled or smoked.

3

The prostate

Alarm over prostate cancer has made the prostate almost synonymous with men's health in recent years. Prostate cancer is the leading cause of cancer deaths in men over 55, and the second most common cause of all male cancer deaths after lung cancer. It affects one in 12 men and the number of new cases is expected to treble over the next 20 years.

Exactly why is not known, nor is the exact cause of prostate problems but, while it is known to run in families, a western diet (high in fat and low in vegetables) may be a trigger. Japanese men have a much lower rate of prostate cancer but when they move to America, and start eating a western diet, their risk of developing the disease becomes the same as American men within two generations.

Other theories as to causes include high levels of the male sex hormone testosterone, and an imbalance between oestrogen and testosterone. This can also be affected by diet, and a prostate-friendly diet is covered in more detail further on in this chapter. Some research work has linked prostate cancer (and other conditions, see Chapter 2) with lack of vitamin D caused by lack of sunlight, as it was found that the further men lived from the equator, the more the incidence of prostate cancer increased.

Chinese research has also shown that prostate cancer is more likely in men who live in cities rather than in the country, and suggests industrial pollution as a likely cause, with the chemical cadmium as a prime suspect.

Prostate cancer, however, accounts for a relatively small proportion of prostate problems, which are more likely the older a man gets and which include benign prostatic hyperplasia, or enlargement of the prostate, and prostatitis, or inflammation of the prostate.

What is the prostate?

The prostate gland, usually described as being about the size and shape of a walnut, is part of the male reproductive system and its growth and function are controlled by various hormones, the most important of which is the male sex hormone testosterone. Found below the bladder and above the base of the penis, it helps nourish the sperm and aid fertility though its full range of functions is not fully understood.

The prostate produces secretions which help keep semen healthy and fluid, so enabling sperm to move more easily and making fertilization of the female egg more likely. Among other things, the prostate secretes sugars along with nutrients such as zinc to help maintain optimal semen health.

Warning signs

The main warning sign that all may not be well with the prostate is difficulty in passing water, as changes in the prostate narrow the urethra, the tube which carries urine from the bladder. This may take a variety of forms including:

- having to wait before the flow of urine starts
- having to pass water urgently, i.e. being unable to wait
- getting up at night to urinate
- difficulty or pain on urination
- urine flow that stops and starts
- feeling of not emptying the bladder completely after urination.

Different diseases of the prostate have various symptoms, which are explained in the sections which follow, but it is important that your partner consults his doctor about any abnormality relating to urination, however minor.

Benign prostatic hyperplasia (BPH)

As the name suggests, benign prostatic hyperplasia (BPH) is a benign or non-cancerous condition and happens when the prostate gland slowly enlarges – although the prostate gland does enlarge naturally with age. The main cause of prostate symptoms, it is far more common than prostate cancer, affecting around 50 per cent of all men at 60, and 80 per cent of men at age 80.

The most common sign of an enlarged prostate is, as described in the box 'Warning signs' above, difficulty in passing urine. This may be difficulty in starting to urinate, a weak flow or one that stops and starts, having to pass water urgently, more often or at night, passing water with effort or discomfort, or dribbling.

The exact cause is not known but various factors have been implicated, especially the male hormone testosterone, which is broken down into dihydrotestosterone (DHT) in the prostate. It may also run in families.

Your partner should consult his doctor if he has any of the above symptoms as BPH can impact a man's quality of life.

Paul, 53, hated having to be aware of everything he drank, for example before bedtime or before going out. He also disliked the social implications such as making sure he knew where the nearest loo was on a visit or outing – he found it embarrassing and degrading. Like many men with BPH, he was also more reluctant to have sex because of his distressing symptoms, and was generally worried about the implications of BPH for his health. Paul's doctor suggested Paul try saw palmetto, which Paul found very helpful (see below).

As well as providing reassurance, a visit to the doctor can also exclude the possibility of more serious disease such as prostate cancer, and prevent complications which are potentially serious, such as kidney damage resulting from trapped urine. His doctor may not prescribe any drugs because the prostate does not necessarily increase in size, and meanwhile other measures can be taken. As noted, Paul's doctor recommended saw palmetto (see next section), while he can also try other measures such as dietary changes (see 'Prostate-friendly diet' below).

If drugs are prescribed these may include alpha-blockers which relax the muscle in the prostate and relieve pressure on the urethra, anti-spasmodic drugs, and 5-alpha-reductase inhibitors which block production of dihydrotestosterone, slowing down the rate at which the prostate is enlarging. (Consult your doctor if you and your partner are planning a pregnancy before taking these drugs.) In more severe cases, surgery may be recommended.

Saw palmetto and other natural remedies

Saw palmetto, a small, palm-like plant, grows in the sand dunes along the Atlantic and Caribbean coasts, and has long been known as a herb which has a therapeutic effect on the bladder and prostate – indeed, one name for it is 'the plant catheter'. Native Americans and early American settlers used the berries to treat problems in the urinary tract, genitals and reproductive system, and it is widely used today to treat prostate problems in Germany and other European countries, Canada and America, and the UK. *The Journal of the American Medical Association* reviewed several clinical trials of saw palmetto and concluded that saw palmetto appeared to improve urinary tract symptoms by about 25 per cent, while men taking saw palmetto were twice as likely to experience improvements as those who were taking a placebo.

Saw palmetto is believed to help maintain prostate health by balancing oestrogen levels. It also helps prevent testosterone from converting into dihydrotestosterone, the hormone believed to cause prostate cells to multiply, leading to an enlarged prostate. The berries also have a reputation as a tonic and aphrodisiac, and are believed to work on the sex hormones.

One American study of middle-aged men with bladder problems found that those who took the herb felt better after six months than did those who took a placebo (although the study also showed the herb did not live up to its anecdotal reputation as an aphrodisiac!). However, your man should not take saw palmetto for treatment of any urinary symptoms without the advice of his doctor.

Available from specialist health stores, saw palmetto can be taken in dried form or drops, or as a tincture. It is supposed to be especially effective for the prostate when taken with chopped nettle root. Chop a couple of handfuls of fresh nettle root, place in a container and cover with saw palmetto tincture. Leave for two weeks, shaking from time to time, then strain and bottle. Take a teaspoon three times a day.

The effects of saw palmetto may take a few weeks to be felt, but it has no significant side effects (although if you decide to try it too, you should not do so if you are pregnant). As with all herbal remedies, it is wise to seek your doctor's advice before starting any course of treatment.

Evening primrose oil is a source of essential fatty acid gammalinolenic acid (GLA) which can slow down prostate enlargement. It may also help a range of other problems from dry skin and acne to irritability and post-viral fatigue.

Rye pollen tablets are another natural remedy for prostate problems, and have a reputation for being especially helpful for chronic non-bacterial prostatitis, although you should allow three to six months for full improvement. Or look for supplements which contain quercetin, a bioflavonoid found naturally in onions and green tea.

Other treatments which some men have found effective include **acupuncture, relaxation techniques and counselling**.

Prostatitis

Prostatitis is infection or inflammation of the prostate which can happen any time to anyone but tends to be more common between 25 and 45. It can take different forms, for example it may be chronic, that is, long-term; or acute, that is, one recent episode. Symptoms vary but may include typical signs of infection such as fevers, sweating and chills, pain and difficulty on urination, having to urinate often or more urgently, aches and pains in the lower back, lower abdomen, thighs and/or genitals, pain on ejaculation, blood in the semen, and infection and swelling of the testes.

Acute bacterial prostatitis is a sudden infection, usually caused by bacteria spreading from the intestines or travelling up the urethra. This form of prostatitis is characterized by a sudden illness with high fever, pain in the lower back and beneath the testicles, and by quite marked symptoms when passing urine.

Chronic prostatitis is when a bacterial infection keeps returning, and symptoms may be less severe than for acute bacterial prostatitis.

Chronic non-bacterial prostatitis is when the prostate becomes inflamed although there appear to be no bacteria present. Most common between 30 and 50, it may be due to problems with emptying the bladder although the condition is not fully understood. The most common symptoms are pain in the testicles, penis or rectum, low backache, pain on passing water, having to urinate often, and discharge from the urethra.

Prostatodynia is a related condition where men suffer symptoms of prostatitis but without any obvious inflammation of the prostate. It is common, accounting for around a third of all men with chronic symptoms of prostatitis. Some experts believe it has a mental component and may be a psychosexual condition; others feel there may be a physical cause such as irritation of the nerves supplying the prostate gland.

Prostatitis, though sometimes difficult to diagnose, can be investigated by means of urine and blood tests, rectal examination, and if necessary biopsy, or removing a piece of the prostate for closer examination under the microscope. Treatment consists of antibiotics and painkillers, especially anti-inflammatories such as ibuprofen.

Cancer of the prostate

Cancer of the prostate seems to run in families – if a man's father or brother has had it, his risk of developing it is around three times greater than normal. Rare in men under 45, the risks rise with age. Often symptomless in the early stages, prostate cancer can cause urinary problems if the tumour starts to press on the urethra, such as difficulty in passing urine, passing urine more frequently, especially at night, pain on passing urine, blood in the urine. Any of these symptoms should result in a visit to the GP, although they may well be for benign reasons.

Unfortunately, prostate cancer can spread, causing symptoms such as weight loss, tiredness, blood in the urine or sperm, and pain in the bones of the pelvis, legs and especially the lower back. However, prostate cancer is slow growing and many older men die of other causes first. Treatment varies depending on how far the cancer has advanced and whether it has spread beyond the prostate gland or not.

Prostate cancer depends on testosterone in order to grow, so some treatments focus on controlling this hormone, especially in the early stages of the cancer. Testosterone is made in the testicles in response to chemical signals from the brain, and drugs can be used to influence this process. Hormonal treatment using tablets or injections to reduce or block testosterone may shrink the cancer and can control it for many years. Unfortunately, there are side effects such as impotence, low sex drive and hot flushes.

Another option is to remove the whole prostate gland if the tumour is small (a radical prostatectomy). It carries a risk of impotence and a lesser one of incontinence, although improvements in surgical techniques mean that these complications are less common than they used to be.

Other types of surgery include TURP (transurethral resection of the prostate) which removes any prostate tissue which is blocking the urethra, although it may not remove all the cancer cells. Some men suffer erection difficulties and retrograde ejaculation afterwards. Occasionally, surgery is also used to remove the inner part of the testicles (orchidectomy) to help control the amount of testosterone in the body. Again, while effective in up to 80 per cent of cases, this produces similar side effects (hot flushes and impotence) as well as psychological and emotional ones.

Radiotherapy may also be used to shrink the prostate gland, using carefully calculated radiation beams, or small, radioactive beads which are inserted into the tumour to release radiation slowly over a period of time. This internal radiotherapy, or brachytherapy, can be as effective as surgery. Side effects vary – some people find them minimal, while others may experience diarrhoea, bleeding and rectal discomfort, as well as problems with erections and continence.

(For further details on prostate cancer and its treatment, read *Coping Successfully with Prostate Cancer* by Dr Tom Smith, Sheldon Press 2002.)

Maintaining prostate health

Following the general advice on diet, exercise and lifestyle in this book will help keep your man in optimal health and protect against a wide range of diseases including prostate disease.

- If he has prostate cancer in the family – for example, a father, brother or uncle who developed the disease at a relatively early age, he should ask his GP about screening with blood tests.
- He should also go to his doctor for any minor symptoms related to passing urine. Although only a small proportion of these turn out to be prostate cancer, the earlier prostate cancer is detected, the more likelihood there is of a cure.
- If he is receiving treatment for any prostate condition and his condition changes, visit your GP at once rather than waiting for your next appointment.
- If he smokes, make giving up a priority – if prostate cancer develops, smoking can make it spread more quickly. Nicotine can also cause muscle spasm, triggering prostatodynia (a similar condition to prostatitis), or making it worse.
- Cut down on alcohol and caffeine.
- Encourage him to take up some form of relaxation – take up a new hobby, join a support group, consider complementary therapies.
- Regular exercise is important to help prevent prostate congestion. Avoid violent exercise when the bladder is full as any urine which spills over into the gland can cause inflammation.
- For prostatodynia, try sitting in a warm to hot bath for half an hour as some studies suggest that warming the gland may speed up the body's natural healing process.
- Identify possible triggers of non-bacterial prostatitis, such as spicy foods, nicotine, smoking and caffeine. If stress is a trigger, try some relaxation techniques.
- Avoid drinking large volumes of liquids at any one time, and avoid drinks altogether before going to bed.
- Suggest he try yoga – certain yoga positions may strengthen the prostate, help with weight loss, and boost general energy.

Prostate-friendly diet

There is now much emphasis on the right diet for prostate health. The traditional diet in Japan, which has a much lower rate of prostate cancer than the UK or America, is low in fat, especially saturated fat, whereas in the United States, areas with the highest consumption of animal fats and dairy produce are also the areas with the highest rates of prostate cancer. Studies have singled out red meat as a particular culprit. It is thought that animal fats may influence hormones and may also block the body's ability to absorb vitamin A, which may protect against cancer.

The traditional eastern diet is high in vegetables, especially coloured ones which contain antioxidant vitamins E, C and betacarotene. These all help destroy free radicals and so protect against cancer and heart disease. It also focuses on rice, soy products, fish, legumes, grains and cruciferous plants (members of the cabbage and turnip families including kohlrabi and Chinese leaves). These contain plant hormones such as isoflavonoids and phytoestrogens which, eaten in sufficient quantities, help balance male hormones and protect against prostate disease.

- Cut down on saturated fat, especially in red meat, animal fats, butter, mayonnaise, and cut down on milk and dairy produce. Use low-fat milk and cheese, and other products (salad dressing, coleslaw).
- Ensure he eats more essential fatty acids such as nuts and seeds, especially pumpkin, which are a traditional male sexual tonic and a home remedy for prostate problems. Other sources of fatty acids include sunflower seeds, linseed or evening primrose oil (see above, 'Saw palmetto and other natural remedies').
- Buy organic meat and dairy products where possible to avoid foods with a high hormone content.
- Ensure he eats more fresh fruit and vegetables. Apart from anything else, these contain fibre which helps flush excess male hormones out of the system, as well as preventing constipation and prostate congestion.
- Increase the family's intake of soya products such as soya beans, tofu and soya flour, as soya helps balance hormone levels. Soya foods contain phytoestrogens, antioxidants, natural cancer-fighters, and other substances which may have a protective effect. Soya beans can be used in casseroles and salads, while soya flour can be used in just about anything – from pancakes and scones to thickening sauces. Look for products which state they have not been genetically modified.

- Swedish research has found that the omega-3 oils in oily fish can help prostate health. Tins are a convenient way of dealing with this – for example, mashed sardine or mackerel on toast, with paprika and lemon juice to taste.
- Include whole grains in his diet, especially rye.
- The minerals zinc and selenium are important for prostate health. If he wants to take zinc supplements, he may be better off consulting his doctor first, as too much zinc can cause stomach upsets. Generally, too, nutrients are thought to have more value when consumed in their source food. Zinc-rich foods include oysters and other shellfish or pine nuts and pumpkin seeds, oatmeal, whole grain products, meat, nuts, milk, eggs and cheese. Sources of selenium include broccoli, mushrooms, molasses, cabbage, garlic, wholegrains, nuts, and seafood such as tuna, oysters and herring.
- Encourage weight loss – fat is a good home for hormones and can trigger hormonal imbalances. (See Chapter 5, 'The inner man', for more on being overweight and how to tackle it.)

4
Fitness

Being a couch potato is one of the biggest threats to men's health today. Few men now start their day by hewing down a tree for fuel and taking the cows to pasture. In the face of a global tide of obesity, decreased physical activity is the factor repeatedly identified as paving the way to 'affluent' diseases such as heart disease, cancers and diabetes.

This is not just in 'developed' countries such as Europe and the USA – obesity is rising in some poorer societies, too. While it is important to resist the so-called 'McDonaldization' of world diet – that is, growing trends towards high fat diets – low levels of physical activity remain a massive threat to health.

In England, for example, only 11 per cent of men (and just 4 per cent of women) meet the most vigorous activity level suggested by the government, while only around a third of men are active enough to give themselves some protection against heart disease.

Partly because of these low activity levels, fitness levels are also low. Around one-third of men (and two-thirds of women) cannot walk up a gradual slope (a 5 per cent gradient) without becoming breathless, and having to stop. Even walking on the level is severe exertion for a large proportion of older people – 45 per cent of men (and 79 per cent of women) aged 65–74 are not fit enough to sustain continuous, normal walking on the level.

Most vigorous activity is achieved through sport and exercise during leisure time – only 4 per cent of men (and 1 per cent of women) engage in vigorous activity at work, whereas about 30 per cent of men (and 20 per cent of women) engage in at least some vigorous sport or recreation, most commonly walking and swimming. But, even though many men exercise or play sport regularly, this still leaves a large number who are not active enough to make a difference to their health.

In fact, 'couch potato-itis' creates as big a risk of heart disease as smoking a pack of cigarettes every day. Being inactive has also been linked to a higher risk of stroke, diabetes, colon cancer, osteoporosis, anxiety, depression, memory loss and low self-esteem. The good news is that it is never too late to start exercising, and gym membership is not compulsory – even increasing your activity by small amounts is beneficial. According to the US Center for Disease Control and the American College of Sports Medicine, just 30 minutes' moderate exercise a day three times a week provides major health benefits; and the 30 minutes of exercise does not have to be taken in a chunk, but can be broken up into sessions of at least 10 minutes throughout the day.

The benefits of exercise

As well as halving the risk of CHD, exercise has time and again been shown to help combat several problems including high blood pressure, stroke and diabetes. Weight-bearing exercise also helps prevent osteoporosis, or fragile bones, usually thought to affect women but which also affects one in 12 men. Regular exercise can also increase bowel activity and so reduce the bloating associated with irritable bowel syndrome. And of course it is incomparable when it comes to helping to lose weight.

On the mental side, exercise improves concentration, mood, sleep and sex drive, and is a highly effective way of dealing with stress and frustration. Studies have shown that it is a powerful anti-depressant – physical activity increases levels of neurotransmitters such as serotonin, which influence the areas of the brain that control mood.

Exercise also reduces stress. In one study, unfit male students were asked to spend ten weeks taking part in an aerobic fitness programme, a relaxation programme, or a discussion group. They were then asked to take part in a stressful competition. The men in the exercise group not only performed better in the test but also experienced much less anxiety, depression and fatigue following the competition than the men in the other two groups.

The gym factor

'Gym' seems to be a magic word or mantra which has acquired a hold over the imagination of many who equate health and fitness. Essential though exercise is to help beat obesity, boost strength and promote healthy bones, it is worth remembering that it is part of a healthy lifestyle, not the only factor in it. The 'gym mentality' does need to be balanced by a broader approach to healthy living which includes not smoking and eating a healthy diet.

These days there is increasing emphasis on the fact that you do not have to go to the gym to achieve results. It is possible to get fit by increasing the amount of exercise you include in your daily life. Just leaving the car at home for a month would make a major difference to many.

Of those who do join a gym, 60 per cent give up less than six months after paying their registration fee. This said, a gym can be a good investment in your health – some people benefit from making their exercise a social event, while it also provides a chance for you both to exercise if you take out joint or family membership. Gyms also offer up-to-the-minute equipment which would be expensive and awkward to have at home, as well as qualified personnel to advise on fitness or offer instruction.

The standard of gyms and health clubs can vary enormously and it is worth visiting a few before making your choice. Factors to bear in mind include:

- interest – is he really interested in working out at a gym or would he – and you – be better off joining a tennis club or paying for skiing lessons?
- location – is it near your home or place of work?
- price – will he (and/or you) use it enough to make it worthwhile?
- availability – how busy is it at peak times such as after work?
- facilities – some gyms do not offer all facilities, for example a swimming pool, so this is worth checking before joining;
- safety – does the gym offer a medical examination before you join?
- qualifications – are qualified instructors (RSA, YMCA or NVQ certificate) available to offer individual supervision and instruction if need be?

- standards – is it affiliated to the Fitness Industry Association?
- hygiene and ventilation – are general standards of these good?

The 'Adonis complex'

The so-called 'Adonis complex' – a fixation with getting fit that can endanger male health – has been explored by US and UK psychologists concerned about the way some men equate masculinity and success with being muscular. The 'Adonis complex' is a term used by some psychologists to describe men who suffer body-image and eating disorders. Just as some people with anorexia may see themselves as 'fat' even when pitifully thin, so some men may be prone to an altered self-image.

One typical disorder is body dysmorphic disorder (in which a man believes that a certain part of his body, like his shoulders, is defective); similarly, there is also muscle dysmorphia (in which men who are very muscular still see themselves as scrawny and small). So, despite the massive increase in male obesity, some men who are desperate to 'get into shape' may go on highly selective diets, or be at risk of anorexic behaviour.

Estimates of men with eating disorders vary, but it is believed that up to 10 per cent of those with anorexia, bulimia and binge eating disorder are men. Experts agree that the problem has increased dramatically in recent years – or, has received more publicity. There is also the possibility that numbers are higher than this but that sufferers remain uncounted and invisible. Many men do not seek treatment, as eating disorders are seen as a totally female province – despite the fact that the case of an anorexic male was one of the first published case histories in medical literature more than 300 years ago.

There are many possible reasons for the increase in eating and body-image disorders among men – above all, advertising. Magazines and TV commercials, even video games, portray an impossibly ideal male body which is used to sell a wide variety of commodities. As with images of women, these airbrushed images are aggressive and unrealistic, showing ever leaner and more muscular pictures of men.

Other reasons for eating and body-image disorders may include previous trauma, or a very pressurized family background, for example with parents who expect too much of their children, especially in terms of athleticism or fitness. As with women, food can be a way of dealing with depression, loneliness and other negative feelings. Runners and weight lifters also seem to have a higher risk of developing eating disorders, according to an American survey, as do men who take part in competitive sports where body shape and size are important (gymnastics, ice skating, dance and wrestling). Eating disorders are just as dangerous to health in men as in women, and may develop into other conditions including heart disease and pancreatitis (a disease of the pancreas). Treatments for eating disorders typically involve some type of cognitive behaviour therapy or psychotherapy.

How to help

- Be alert for any warning signs that your partner may be taking his training too seriously, such as preoccupation with his body, weight and shape; restricting the amounts or types of foods eaten (e.g. eating no fat or eating only vegetables); feeling ashamed of his body (e.g. refusing to take a jacket off on a warm day for fear of showing his 'thin' shoulders).
- If you suspect your partner has an eating disorder, persuade him to visit the family doctor and accompany him – many GPs may not diagnose an eating disorder in a man. Ask for a referral to a psychotherapist who specializes in the treatment of these disorders.
- Contacting a nutritionist or dietician (see 'Useful addresses') may also help him towards better eating habits.
- Contact a support group (see 'Useful addresses').

How fit is he?

A brisk walk, climbing up the stairs at the station, running after a small runaway child, can all tell whether he is averagely fit or whether exercise leaves him puffing. Checking his pulse before and after exercise is a good way to test fitness. To test a resting pulse, place two or three fingers over the wrist or press gently into the side of the neck, and count for one minute. The average for a reasonably fit man is 72 beats a minute but can range between 50 and 90 depending on fitness. The lower it is, the more fit he is likely to be. If your man is under 40 and has a pulse over 85, you should be concerned about fitness; in older men, a pulse rate over 90 should give cause for concern. Test the resting pulse a few times a day after sitting quietly for 10 minutes to get a true overall picture.

See how quickly your heartbeat returns to normal after a period of exercise – the quicker it does, the fitter you are. Next time you exercise, keep measuring your pulse every 30 seconds afterwards and see how long it takes to return to normal. There is no set time for this to happen but the quicker it happens the fitter you are, and you can keep using this measurement as a general indication of how fit you are.

Men in their 20s
Above 102 – unfit
Below 75 – fit

Men in their 30s
Above 104 – unfit
Below 79 – fit

Men in their 40s
Above 106 – unfit
Below 81 – fit

Men in their 50s
Above 108 – unfit
Below 83 – fit

The three classic components of overall fitness and health are stamina, strength and suppleness:

Stamina, or endurance, is the ability to keep on exercising without stopping to rest which depends on how well his heart, lungs, muscles and circulation perform. Stamina is best built up by regular aerobic (needing oxygen) exercise which builds up a healthy heart. It also reduces fat, as it boosts the metabolism not just during the exercise, but even after the exercise has finished.

An easy way for him to build stamina is to take moderate aerobic exercise for at least 30 minutes a day three days a week. This could be brisk walking, swimming, table tennis, golf, dancing, heavy DIY (e.g. mixing cement), digging the garden and heavy housework – anything which makes his heart beat faster than usual, raises the heartbeat and leaves him feeling slightly warm and slightly out of breath.

As he gets fitter, he can aim to increase his level of exercise to two or three continuous and vigorous 20–30 minute aerobic workouts each week. This level of exercise – which includes running, fast cycling and rowing – provides the optimum health benefits.

Strength is built up by repeated aerobic exercise over a period of time, which basically keeps muscle groups in trim, boosting his metabolism so he burns calories faster, leaving him with more muscle bulk and less fat. It also increases muscle strength, protects against injury, and develops the muscles' lifting and carrying abilities. As the body contains more than 600 muscles, strength is important! The safest and easiest way for him to improve his strength is to use weights machines in a gym.

Suppleness, or flexibility, is the ability to stretch or bend through a wide range of movements. Regular stretching will not only increase his flexibility, it will also help protect him against sports injuries and can leave him feeling relaxed and energized. Yoga and Pilates are great for this.

Sports injuries

There are 29 million sports injuries each year in Britain, the most common ones being sprains and strains of the lower limbs, according to research at Sheffield University. One-third of these are serious enough to result in medical treatment or to affect normal activities. Half of all tennis players develop tennis elbow (a painful inflammation caused by over-use of the muscles around the elbow joint). And, rugby, judo and other contact sports can transmit scrumpox, a rash caused by bacteria, viruses or fungi.

Five major causes of sports injuries are:

- not warming up properly;
- overtraining or not training properly – frequent and intensive training can also lower immunity and resistance to disease;
- poor equipment, especially footwear – every pound of your weight translates into around four pounds impacting on your knee with every step. Proper footwear acts as a shock absorber;

- not being fit – he should gradually work up to fitness, especially if he has had to stop through injury or illness for a while;
- the environment – harsh surfaces such as pavements, or unfamiliar ground, increase the risk of injury.

To prevent injury, your partner really needs to give his body time to recover from each bout of exercise, especially if he is new to training. Ensure he has a good, well-balanced diet with plenty of vitamin C.

If he does injure himself, apply ice to the area and insist that he rests. Time off the activity may be needed – if in doubt, he should consult his doctor about how long he should avoid the activity for. He should not be encouraged to start again before the set time, to avoid the risk of further or more sustained injury. He should also ask his doctor's advice if either of you is concerned about an injury, as neglected ones can often develop into something worse.

Warming up

Warming up before exercise is vital to prevent sports injuries like torn muscles, and the older he is, the more important it is (although young people can sustain injury too if they neglect this). More warming up is needed in cold weather, and he should allow half an hour for vigorous sports such as football.

Warming up prepares the muscles for more movement by feeding them glucose and oxygen. As the muscle temperature increases – or as they literally 'warm up' – they become more flexible and so he can stretch and move the joints with less risk of injury. Warming up also helps prevent osteoarthritis, a fact of life for many sportsmen.

Some sports people feel that a period of warming down is just as important – but you do not have to go for a three-mile jog after exercise to cool down. A 15–30 minute walk, depending on the level of exercise you have just been doing, will do.

Sports nutrition

A varied, healthy diet is usually enough for the demands of the averagely fit man.

He should eat before exercise so as not to exercise on an empty stomach, but not too soon, to avoid cramps and indigestion. Leaving two to three hours after eating can also lessen the likelihood of stomach cramp or stitch.

A light meal or snack (plus drink – see the box below, 'Staying hydrated') two to three hours beforehand is ideal. Carbohydrates (wholegrain sandwich or toast, baked potato, pasta, dried or fresh fruit or bagels) are usually recommended as they are digested more quickly than high-fat or high-protein meals, so providing the body with glucose (sugar) for more sustained energy.

If he is training seriously or does a lot of heavy physical exertion, he should eat a diet rich in complex carbohydrates, keep fat intake to a minimum, and include oily fish, nuts and seeds. If he does want to pursue sports nutrition further, read *The Complete Book of Men's Health* by Dr Sarah Brewer (see 'Further reading'), or seek advice from a sports dietician.

Staying hydrated

It is important to drink enough fluids before and during exercise as dehydration is a major cause of fatigue in exercise and can also cause cramp. On average, a man sweats around a litre an hour during exercise, nearly two and a half in hot weather. Thirst is not a reliable guide to how much fluid he needs, as by the time he feels thirsty he may already be dehydrated, so he should drink before he feels thirsty.

A good plan is to have one or two glasses of water half an hour before beginning and drink small amounts at regular intervals throughout exercise. He should be especially wary in hot weather.

Water is the best drink. Watch out for high glucose drinks and sports drinks and snack bars which can contain a lot of added sugar. While they may help with an endurance event such as a long run, the extra calories they contain are fattening and can add to fatigue as glucose is absorbed very quickly by the bloodstream – a more sustained source of energy is carbohydrates, complex if possible. The high sugar may cause dehydration by drawing water out of the bloodstream to the stomach to 'dilute' the drink. Alcohol should be avoided straight after exercise as it too is diuretic (i.e. makes you pass water) – as are coffee, tea and cola drinks – he can have a non-alcoholic drink first. Salt tablets usually are not needed unless he is training vigorously in hot weather and is having to drink large amounts to stay hydrated.

If he is training for an hour or more an isotonic sports drink (fluid, electrolytes and 6–8 per cent carbohydrate) is a good choice.

Staying with it

Sad to say, it often takes some serious motivation like a health scare to make people stay with exercise. They do it because they have to. But, for many, plans that seemed easy in summer may fall by the wayside as it gets colder or darker, or work demands overtime, or the fitness plan does not seem to be losing the weight. Most people abandon their fitness regime within the year. But it is possible to stick with it.

Doing exercise because he feels he ought to probably will not work. He is much more likely to stick with it if he is motivated to get fit for himself, and if he finds something he enjoys, which can vary widely, from a solitary cycle ride to a football club or jazz dance.

- Encourage small steps. Leave out his exercise clothes and shoes at the end of the bed or by the front door so they are easily accessible. Even if he just puts them on and potters round the garage, it is still one small step towards exercise and goes a little way towards creating an exercise mentality!

- Accompany him on a run for the first five minutes. By the time you have both run back, that is ten minutes – long enough for the exercise to have kicked in and warmed you up so that you feel ready to continue.
- Glide over setbacks. There will be days when he is too tired or busy to exercise, but this need not stop him getting on with it again the next day. Hard-gained fitness does not vanish in a day or two, so encourage him to keep at it as a long-term plan.
- Having clear-cut goals will make him more likely to stick with it, for example, wanting to lose a stone in six months' time, or get fit for a holiday, or increase the amount of daily exercise by ten minutes. Aimless exercise is demoralizing.
- Write down successes. Keep an exercise diary in which to record progress such as weight loss, length of exercise time, number of calories the calorie counter at the gym records, and so on. Focusing on his successes will boost his self-confidence and make it easier to think of himself as someone who can exercise and lose weight.

Get more exercise into his life

He needs to take any opportunity that offers physical activity. Even five minutes walking at a time, a few times a day, makes a difference. Encourage him to:

- take up a former sport he enjoyed
- take advantage of any sporting facilities at work, or any discounts to clubs or gyms
- take out family membership of a health club
- go swimming, walking or dancing with you
- walk to the shops (carrying the bags back counts, too). Or at least park at the far end of the supermarket carpark
- walk to the school to drop off or pick up the children
- pick up the children by foot from other activities such as guides or choir – it teaches them habits of activity, too
- take the children to the park and play actively with them

- teach the children swimming, tennis or some other sport, and exercise with them (they need the physical activity too). Look for fun activities such as rollerblading or skateboarding, and they will love the activity and the company
- buy a bike, or bikes for the family, or join a local cycle club
- explore ways of getting to work that could involve more activity, such as cycling to the next train station instead of getting the train at your nearest station
- use his lunch hour at work for a brisk walk, a swim or a run round the park
- walk or cycle to work or on short journeys such as to the library or post office
- get off the bus or tube a stop early and walk
- take up a physical hobby such as gardening – if he starts a kitchen garden, he may be more likely to consume the fruits of his labours, so adding to his nutritional health too!

Getting the most from exercise

Both you and your partner should consult a doctor before beginning an exercise programme if you are over 40, have heart or joint problems, have not done any exercise recently, are very overweight, smoke, have a family history of heart disease before 40, or are under medical treatment for any condition.

He should not exercise if he has a cold, sore throat, temperature, cough or other sign of infection, as increasing his heart rate through strenuous exertion when he has a virus can cause harm or result in serious damage such as inflammation of the heart (myocarditis). So, allow a few days off to ensure full recovery.

He is more likely to stick at it if he chooses a time to exercise that suits him. Studies have shown that evening exercisers are more likely to stick to their routines for longer and this may be due to psychological factors, for example that people feel entitled to relax after the day's work is done. Going too early may leave him tired out for the day especially in the early stages of fitness, while going too late may leave him too wired to sleep. Late afternoon or early evening may be a better time to go – trial and error will probably reveal the best time for him.

5

The inner man – diet, obesity and digestive problems

Take a look at the average British male when he strips off on holiday and you could be forgiven for thinking that there had been no health education in the UK for the last 100 years or so. Obesity reigns – not just among middle-aged men with the classic beer belly, but among young teenagers and even children.

The majority of men in England are now either fat or obese, according to a government report on obesity, which has tripled in men over the past two decades. According to the report, around 60 per cent of men are overweight and 17 per cent clinically obese. Obesity is now seen as a serious health problem which needs urgent tackling. Many obese men will not live out their full span of years – being obese can reduce life expectancy by as much as nine years, while around 30,000 people a year die in the UK as a result of conditions linked with obesity. Coronary heart disease causes 270,000 heart attacks each year in the UK, of which the British Heart Foundation estimates that 28,000 are directly attributable to obesity. Obesity puts a strain on all the inner parts of the body – heart, frame, organs (why this chapter is called 'The inner man'). Being overweight goes much deeper than vanity. Along with inactivity, it is one of the biggest threats to male health today.

The good news is that it can be tackled, and losing even a little weight has positive effects on health. According to National Audit Office figures, sustained weight loss of 5–10kg (11–22lbs) can reduce the chances of fatal heart disease by 9 per cent, and can cut the chances of cancer by more than a third. However, yet again it may be up to you to take the lead. Men are often not as concerned about their weight as women are, and the majority of men still tend to leave shopping, food and cooking choices to their partners.

What causes obesity

In a society dominated by the car and the TV, lack of physical activity is a major factor in being overweight. A high-fat diet does play havoc with weight (and health in general), but lack of physical activity cannot be underestimated in creating obesity (see Chapter 4 on 'Fitness').

There are other influences. Most people gain more weight with age, especially round the abdomen – the familiar creeping weight gain over the years, especially if he smokes or regularly drinks a lot. Hereditary influences do play a part in an estimated 35–40 per cent of people. Genes may influence appetite, levels of activity, food preferences, and how and why they eat. Equally, though, environment – usually parental influence – plays a part in all these.

However, genes do not explain the surge of obesity in recent years. Nor do theories such as that obese people lack leptin, a body chemical which helps control appetite. These may be factors for some people but, overall, lifestyle, including a high-fat diet, is the biggest influence.

Why obesity is bad for him

The health risks of obesity are multiple. Obesity is the biggest cause of cancer apart from smoking and, in particular, obese men are at increased risk from cancer of the colon, rectum and prostate.

Other risks of being obese include diabetes, heart disease, high blood pressure, arthritis, stroke, varicose veins, kidney disorders and fertility problems such as low sperm count, low libido and subfertility. Obesity can also worsen conditions such as snoring and sleep apnoea (interrupted breathing during sleep), as well as asthma. The strain on the back, and on other joints such as knees and hips, can also cause problems.

Fat around the abdomen (the 'beer belly') can be a particular health risk. 'Apple-shaped' men are at greater risk of coronary heart disease, stroke, high blood pressure, atherosclerosis, high cholesterol, gallstones and diabetes than 'pear-shaped' men who have fat more on the hips and rest of the body. This may be related to different types of metabolism which process fat in different ways.

Regular exercise does have a significant impact on this, even if not much exercise has been done before.

The psychological and emotional effects of too much weight have to be taken into account, too. While men may not be as concerned as women about excess weight, they are not indifferent. Being overweight saps energy, confidence and sex drive.

The way out of all this is determination but, with men, it often takes some crisis to precipitate a change. Too often, the man on a 'diet' is one who has been told he has to lose weight for the sake of his health.

Charles was told he had to have a kidney transplant but only if he could lose some weight – at 23 stone, he was seriously clinically obese, and the operation would be too dangerous in his present state. He was also developing heart problems, and had suffered high blood pressure for years. He also had severe sleep apnoea and was permanently tired.

John had no overt health problems but there was heart disease in the family and he felt he was becoming alarmingly breathless on relatively little exertion such as climbing the station stairs on the way to work in the morning. At 15 stone, he was three stone heavier than he had been when he had married. His doctor told him he had asthma directly caused by his excess weight.

Both men took action (with the help of their wives). John rejected the diagnosis of asthma but started to take more physical activity and watched what he ate. Charles took the – for men – drastic step of joining a slimming club (see the box, 'Slimming clubs and other support', below).

Get him moving

Today's lifestyle forces us to be sedentary, so fight it. Make it a priority to get more physical activity into his life – maybe yours, too, if you do not already do as it can only benefit you

---

49

as well. Even if not much weight is lost, it will still benefit your overall health. American research has found that moderately or very fit men had a lower risk of dying from any cause than men with low fitness levels, despite their weight. If he has a medical condition, is very overweight, or is over 40 and has not done any exercise for a while, he should check with his doctor before taking up an exercise programme.

For suggestions on how to encourage him to be more physically active, see Chapter 4 on 'Fitness'.

Weight management – the 5 per cent factor

Losing just 5 per cent of his total body weight can have a substantial and long-term positive effect on his health. We do live in a 'slimming' culture that demands instant results, but there is increasing recognition that losing small amounts of weight at a time is valuable, and the notion of long-term healthy eating more effective than 'slimming'. It takes time to change eating and exercise habits, and diets are notoriously hard to keep to. The majority of people who lose a lot of weight put it back on within the first year, so small losses may be easier to achieve and keep up than sudden large ones. He can always aim to lose another 5 per cent after that.

Trying to lose weight too quickly tends not to work, because the body interprets this as starvation and goes into survival mode, slowing down its metabolism by up to 30 per cent, and holding on to its fat stores. Your man may also lose more muscle – but, if he starts eating more again, he tends to regain the fat but not the muscle. The trick is to think long-term. For weight management to be effective, aim for gradual changes in eating behaviour (and exercise), planning to lose no more than 1–2lbs (0.5–1kg) a week.

How to help

Getting your man to lose weight may be an area where you have to be as cunning as the serpent and as gentle as the dove. Carrying the message too stridently is likely to be counterproductive. Your man may enjoy comfort food, or have traditional favourites, or dislike change in eating habits, or he may simply expect to eat what he likes at the end of a hard day's work. However, there are several ways in which you can increase both his awareness of what he eats, and his healthy eating habits.

- Measure his waist – the risk of CHD increases if it is over 94cm (37 inches), as apple-shape obesity is linked with atherosclerosis. Ask him to exhale slowly. Then measure his waist 1cm below the tummy button – he should not be holding his stomach muscles tightly in:
  under 94cm – healthy
  94–101cm – increased health risk
  over 101cm – much greater health risk.
- Try and get him to eat a healthy breakfast. It takes seconds to whizz up pancakes in the blender, made with an equal mix of oatmeal, soya flour and wholegrain flour, along with an egg white and skimmed milk. Or, wholegrain toast, cereal, raw or cooked oats, fruit, low-fat milk or yoghurt, or baked beans, all will fill him up, kickstart his metabolism and get his blood sugar balanced for a good start to the day. Breakfast eaters tend to be slimmer and have lower cholesterol levels than those who do not eat it (they also catch fewer infections such as colds, according to research at the University of Cardiff).
- Plan small changes one at a time. For example, start the evening meal with a homemade vegetable soup, again made quickly in the blender, which immediately increases vegetable intake, also boosting his intake of fibre, vitamins and minerals, and filling him up so he may eat less of the rest of the meal. Then tackle something else, such as making his packed lunch healthier.
- Look for ways of cooking family favourites so they are less fattening: use low-fat milk, yoghurt or low-fat fromage frais instead of full-fat milk and cream; lemon juice, mustard and yoghurt instead of mayonnaise or salad dressing; mix lentils with minced turkey for lasagne or shepherd's pie instead of using fattier lamb or beef mince; use tinned tomatoes instead of creamy sauces for pasta sauces; and so on. Use low-fat cooking methods – grill, bake, microwave, barbecue, stir-fry, steam, chargrill.

51

- Plan your shopping – go to a small supermarket or shop online so you are not tempted by endless aisles of food. Buy plenty of fruit, carrots, celery, etc. for nibbles – not biscuits.
- Have regular meals and keep snacks minimal – this helps control appetite.
- Base meals on complex carbohydrate foods such as wholewheat or grain cereals, bread, rice, potatoes, pasta. These boost levels of serotonin in the brain, raising your mood and making you feel more full. They also boost your metabolic rate which helps burn off more fat.
- Just cutting out alcohol can do wonders for weight reduction.
- Discourage comfort or boredom eating, i.e. in front of the TV.
- You cannot control what he eats at work but you can provide a healthy packed lunch, or suggest healthy choices from the canteen. Many men are genuinely not aware of exactly which foods can be fattening, such as salad dressings, so he may need telling.
- Encourage him to eat more slowly by playing soothing music at meals.
- Suggest he (or you) keep a food diary for a week to learn more about his eating habits.
- Check for food allergies which may sometimes cause fluid retention. If he is not losing as much weight as you think he should be, try cutting out all sugar, alcohol, white flour, dairy products, red meat and eggs for a couple of weeks. For more information on whether food allergies could be causing weight gain, read *The Waterfall Diet* by Linda Lazarides (see 'Further reading').
- If he is overweight or obese, and has a family history of heart disease, high blood pressure or diabetes, it may be worth him asking his GP for a check-up, including diabetes, cholesterol and blood pressure tests.
- Your GP will also be able to advise him if he is not losing any weight after a steady programme of sensible eating and exercise. This might be due to an underlying physical disorder which needs investigation. Treatments for obesity itself include therapy if eating disorders are linked to deep-seated emotional problems; weight-control drugs; and as a last resort, surgery for severely

obese people with serious health risks, who have not been able to lose weight with other approaches, although this can pose other health risks (for example stomach stapling, in which part of the intestine is removed, carries the risk of liver and kidney damage).

Slimming clubs and other support

Slimming clubs tend to be seen as a women-only area, but they do welcome the few men who are brave enough to step through the doors (fewer than one in 100).

> Charles, mentioned above as weighing 23 stone, knew he needed to do something about his weight but originally accompanied his wife to a slimming club, as she wanted to lose 3 stone but was too shy to go on her own. She lost her weight – and Charles, over 18 months – lost a staggering 8 stone. 'It was a bit daunting at first but the ladies were very kind and I'm now being entered as slimmer of the year for our local awards,' says Charles.

Online support may be easier for some men. Good web sites to visit are listed at the end of this book (see 'Useful addresses').
Another alternative is Fatmanslim, the UK's first weight loss programme aimed directly at men, invented by obesity expert Dr Ian Campbell, chairman of the Men's Health Forum which aims to raise awareness of male health (see 'Useful addresses'). Fatmanslim works by persuading men to gradually eat less food, to cut down on saturated fat, snacks and alcohol, and to eat more vegetables. Dr Campbell says that by following his programme, the average beer gut should be trimmed by 4 inches in 12 weeks. He has also worked out that if only one in 200 overweight British men stick with the programme, the weight of the nation would drop by more than 1,000 tonnes! (The kit, costing £84, is available by mail order from FMS Healthcare, Nottingham, UK – see 'Useful addresses'.)

The fat trap

Fat levels are far too high in the average man's diet, accounting for more than 40 per cent of calories, and are a major source of weight gain and raised cholesterol levels. It is recommended that fat makes up less than 30 per cent of his daily intake of calories.

The main fats to avoid are saturated ones, which increase the risk of atherosclerosis, and are mostly found in animal foods, for example fatty meat, cheese, butter, cream. Hydrogenated fats found in fatty processed and fast foods are also saturated fats.

Instead, choose foods rich in essential fatty acids, like healthy omega-3 fats, needed to regulate functions such as blood pressure and clotting. Good sources include oily fish (mackerel, salmon, kippers, trout, sardines), rapeseed oil, soya oil and spread, walnut oils, pumpkin seeds and linseeds, wholegrains, walnuts and sweet potatoes.

In moderation, mono-unsaturated fats are good for blood cholesterol levels. Good sources include olive oil and olive oil-based spreads, rapeseed oil, avocados and most nuts.

Does he need vitamin supplements?

Ideally, the best way to obtain vitamins is from a healthy diet and, for vitamin D, from sunlight or daylight. Eating the foods which contain vitamins gives you the benefit of other nutrients, such as minerals and phytochemicals, as well as fibre, which you do not get when taking the isolated vitamin as a supplement.

Research suggests that men are most likely to have a low intake of some minerals, such as zinc, magnesium, selenium and potassium, and also of vitamin E. The best way to get these is to include more of the foods containing these in his diet.

- **Zinc:** oysters, offal, meat, mushrooms, eggs, wholegrain products (including cereals such as porridge or branded wholegrain cereals); brewer's yeast
- **Magnesium:** brown rice, soybeans, nuts, brewer's yeast, wholewheat flour, legumes

- **Selenium:** wheatgerm, bran, tuna fish, kidneys, onions, tomatoes, broccoli and wholewheat bread
- **Potassium:** fresh fruit and vegetables, especially bananas, dried apricots, pulses, mushrooms, potatoes and spinach
- **Vitamin E:** wheatgerm, soybeans, vegetable oils, broccoli, leafy green vegetables, whole grains, peanuts, eggs

Supplements of specific nutrients are useful if he has to restrict certain foods – for example, if he has a milk allergy, then he might want to consider a calcium supplement to prevent osteoporosis, the fragile bone disease which affects one in 12 men. It is best to take supplements as a complete all-in-one multivitamin and mineral, to prevent imbalances that might be caused by, say, taking large amounts of just one B vitamin; or, consult a nutritional therapist.

Eating disorders

Numbers vary as to how many men suffer eating disorders such as anorexia, bulimia and binge eating, but some estimates put them as high as one in six. Research suggests that eating disorders in men often seem to go hand in hand with abnormal pressure to achieve a 'perfect' body – resulting in what has been termed the 'Adonis complex'. As this tends to happen more often in men very concerned with fitness, this subject is covered more fully in Chapter 4, 'Fitness'. Do read this if you suspect your man has an eating disorder, as it needs to be taken seriously, and can be treated.

Those inner problems

Being obese is a major risk factor for many 'inner' problems, such as diabetes, indigestion, heartburn, ulcers and irritable bowel syndrome. Apart from encouraging him to lose weight, there are other ways you may be able to lessen the discomfort of these conditions, too.

Diabetes

Men are one-and-a-half times more likely than women to get diabetes, which affects around 30 per cent of people in the UK.

Diabetes mellitus (sugar diabetes) is when the pancreas does not produce enough insulin, a hormone which controls glucose levels, absorbing glucose from the bloodstream into the body cells, where it is converted into energy. As a result, diabetics have abnormally high blood glucose levels, which plays havoc with normal body functions. For example, without insulin, muscles waste away because the muscle protein cannot be built up from the high amounts of sugar in the body.

Insulin-dependent diabetes, also known as juvenile or Type 1 diabetes, is the most severe form and is when people cannot produce any insulin of their own and usually appears before 35. It needs early diagnosis and treatment as it has complications and can be life-threatening, causing blindness, kidney failure, heart disease, stroke, nerve damage and impotence.

Non-insulin dependent or Type 2 diabetes, when insulin is produced but not in large enough quantities, usually happens after 40. While insulin may not always be needed for treatment, Type 2 needs treatment just as urgently as Type 1. Paying attention to diet and exercise can, however, be effective in preventing it.

There is concern that many people in the UK may have diabetes and do not know it – the 'missing million'. Do ensure he checks any warning signs with his doctor. These include blurred vision, excessive thirst, frequent urination, fatigue and weakness, itchiness, especially round the genitals, and numbness and tingling in the feet and hands.

What you can do
The more overweight the man, and the less physical activity he does, the greater his risk of diabetes, so try and put some of this chapter's suggestions about weight management into practice. In particular, central body fat (being 'apple shaped') is linked to Type 2 diabetes. Genetic factors and ageing also make some men more likely to get diabetes.

Heartburn

Heartburn is very common and is a painful burning feeling in the breastbone which may be mild or so intense as to be mistaken for a heart attack. People with heartburn may also feel bloated because they swallow air in an unconscious attempt to relieve discomfort.

Heartburn may be caused when stomach acid is regurgitated into the oesophagus, which tends to happen especially if people are overweight. Fizzy drinks such as sparkling mineral water can also raise pressure inside the stomach, while coffee, smoking and alcohol can all cause acid reflux by relaxing the muscular valve which usually stops this acid overflow. Hiatus hernia, when part of the stomach protrudes up into the chest cavity, can also prevent the valve closing properly.

What you can do
- Suggest he eats several small meals a day rather than two or three big ones.
- He should not eat just before going to bed.
- He should cut down on alcohol, particularly neat spirits.
- He must stop smoking.
- Try and identify any specific food which may be causing his heartburn such as rich, fatty or spicy foods, or acidic foods like grapefruit and tomatoes.
- He can avoid bending over, lying down or exercising one hour after eating.
- He can also avoid wearing a tight belt or clothes.
- Let him sleep with extra pillows or put a couple of books under the bed legs at the bed head.
- He can take an antacid immediately after a meal.

See your doctor if these self-help measures do not work. He or she may prescribe a drug which reduces the amount of stomach acid or that tightens the muscular valve. In severe cases, surgery may be needed for hiatus hernia.

Irritable bowel syndrome

Irritable bowel syndrome (IBS), though better known for its impact on women, affects around one in 12 men in the UK, with a range of distressing symptoms including excess wind, pain in the abdomen

57

and constipation and diarrhoea. If any of these are persistent, it is worth him checking them out with his doctor, although it is more likely that his doctor will not find anything definite behind any symptoms. The exact cause of IBS is unknown but stress and lifestyle are major factors. For example, the bowel has receptors for stress hormones such as adrenaline which can cause muscle spasm.

What you can do
- Try more fibre in his diet for a couple of weeks.
- Get him to eat plenty of fresh fruit or buy a juicer to increase his intake.
- Try excluding dairy products from his diet for a few weeks to see if the IBS is due to food intolerance or allergy.
- Avoid using red meat and saturated fats and sugar.
- Avoid frying or roasting food.
- Suggest he cuts down on tea and coffee, which stimulate bowel action.
- Try him on live yoghurt to promote the friendly bacteria *Lactobacillus acidophilus*.
- In cooking, try and use spices known for their digestive powers including aniseed, clove oil, black pepper, parsley and peppermint.
- Get him to drink plenty of water, including herbal teas.
- Encourage him to cut down on stress – see the section on stress in Chapter 8.
- Exercise may help and is an effective stress-buster.
- Smoking, among its other evils, stimulates receptors in the bowel which can contribute to irritation.

Indigestion and ulcers
Indigestion affects twice as many men as women, with symptoms such as bloating, pain, nausea, while peptic ulcer affects twice as many men as women. Once again, he should lose weight and stop smoking. The following suggestions may help in both cases, but if symptoms persist do consult your doctor as there may be an underlying problem. Inform him or her of what remedies you have already tried as well.

What you can do

- Again, he should eat little and often and not late at night.
- He can avoid hot, spicy, fatty foods, mint chocolate and fruit juices, tea, coffee, and alcohol.
- He should take paracetamol rather than aspirin to avoid irritating the stomach.
- Raise the head of your bed with pillows or a support beneath the legs.
- A glass of milk may help ease symptoms.
- For wind, he could try bicarbonate of soda in warm water every hour for three hours (but no longer).
- For indigestion, try an antacid from your pharmacy, or homeopathic remedies such as nux vomica, bryonia and pulsatilla.
- Try the natural herbs suggested for IBS above.

6

The outer man

Dealing with hair and skin problems is important as they may affect a man's well-being and quality of life – some skin problems also have serious implications for his health.

Haircare and loss

Hair loss has been a notoriously emotive subject for men since the days of Samson and probably before. It is normal to lose up to 150 hairs a day, although usually new hair grows within three months. Balding is also usual – male-pattern balding (alopecia androgenetica), the most common type, where hair thins over temples and crown, affects at least two-thirds of all men, while almost 95 per cent of men experience some form of hair loss during their lives. While it tends to be hereditary, testosterone is a factor, affecting the hair follicles so that they fail to produce hair. Diet may also be a factor, as Japanese and Chinese men, as well as having less prostate disease, also have less baldness (see Chapter 3 for details of an eastern diet).

At the extreme end, treatment includes transplants, wigs and drugs (which he will have to pay for himself). Minoxidil (sold as Regaine) is a lotion to be rubbed into the scalp, available from his pharmacist, who should check that he can safely use it as it can have side effects (for instance, he should not use it without medical supervision if he has high blood pressure). It is claimed that it causes regrowth in around 15 per cent of those who use it.

Finasteride (Propecia) is a drug available on private prescription but also has side effects in some, including impotence. He should consult his GP first.

In the rarer cases when balding results from an imbalance of sex hormones, hormonal drugs are available but should only be taken under expert supervision – again, he should consult his doctor.

Sudden hair loss is worth having investigated as it may be caused by a range of conditions including thyroid disease, ringworm, chronic illness, high fever or hormonal imbalance. Anxiety, shock, stress and, sometimes, nutritional deficiencies such as lack of iron can also cause hair loss. 'Medical' balding is known as alopecia areata, and can affect all the hair on the body including eyebrows. While the underlying cause is not always found, the hair does usually eventually grow back.

Finally, the much rarer excess of hair is also worth investigating as it can be caused by tumours of the adrenal cortex or disorders of the pituitary or thyroid gland.

Hair care – what you can do

- Make sure his diet includes enough protein, especially if you are vegan or vegetarian – hair loss or greying can sometimes be due to a poor diet, especially one deficient in protein. Eat iron-rich foods such as liver, eggs and green vegetables.
- A traditional home remedy for balding is sage tea, an infusion made from boiling water and sage leaves, both drunk and rubbed into the scalp.
- Nettle tea is also said to stimulate hair growth as well as cleansing the system and boosting liver function. Steep the tips in boiling water for a few minutes.
- Persuade him to treat his hair gently – most people are far too rough with it. Wet hair is fragile, and should be combed gently, and not rubbed too hard. Blowdrying, overbrushing, and exposure to too much chlorine or sun weaken the hair and cause split ends.
- He should shampoo hair regularly and could massage his scalp to stimulate blood flow (or you could do this). Good oils include rosemary, lavender, sage, cedarwood or ylang ylang.
- A lot of 'dandruff' is caused by too much strong shampoo and not enough rinsing, both of which dry the scalp and result in flaking. It is better to use only a small amount of shampoo (about the size of a 10p piece), then rinse under a shower for several minutes. Instead of using harsh anti-dandruff shampoos, he could try a mild fragrance-free or baby one, plus conditioner.

Acne

Acne is an inflammatory condition that occurs in the tiny hair roots and their oil or sebaceous glands in the skin. It is most common on the face, neck, back and shoulders and may show as inflamed spots or whiteheads and blackheads.

Acne is caused by too much oil which blocks hair follicles, eventually resulting in inflammation. It is related to the dramatic increase in the levels of the sex hormone testosterone in teenage years, although it can persist well after that – around 1 per cent of men at 40 still have acne needing treatment. In most people, however, it clears up on its own.

Contrary to popular myth, acne is not related to cleanliness or diet. Factors which can make it worse include sweating, which can increase follicle blockages, hot, damp weather, oils such as suntan oils or creams, and some clothing such as nylon, polyester or tight clothing.

Mild to moderate acne can often be controlled using over-the-counter preparations, such as creams and lotions containing benzoyl peroxide. (Consult your pharmacist.) If these do not work after a period of two months, or if your condition is more severe, see your doctor who may prescribe antibiotics or drugs such as vitamin A derivatives.

Sunbathing and skin cancer

Exposure to sunlight can be a helpful treatment for acne, but it is important to avoid overexposure as too much strong sun may cause skin cancer. Examine the skin regularly to detect skin cancer which is treatable if caught early, especially if he has a fair complexion, a large number of moles or large moles, or has had cancer in the family. You are in a good position to help as you can examine his back and neck, which of course he cannot see himself!

Warning signs include:
- a change in skin texture and colour
- a mole or blemish that changes in shape, size or colour or starts to bleed

- a sore or ulcer that fails to heal within three weeks
- the sudden appearance of a new mole.

For more on skin cancer see Chapter 2, 'Cancers'.

What you can do

- Try and get him to drink plenty of water, including herbal teas, but not fizzy drinks, tea or coffee.
- He could try electric razors rather than a wet shave.
- Try aromatherapy oils such as bergamot, geranium, lavender and lemon, or herbalist lavender, marigold or elderflower.
- Enough vitamin A, B complex and C, and the mineral zinc, all help skin health. Supplements may help.
- Avoid creams and lotions, or discuss with a doctor or pharmacist.
- While there is no medical evidence that chocolate or sweets make acne worse, some foods may make it worse in some individuals. He could try eliminating processed, sugary and refined foods for a while.
- Getting plenty of daylight may help. Sunlight is thought to improve moderate acne in about 60 per cent of cases. Ultraviolet light treatment can also be used, and a new treatment using red and blue light has been found to be effective at healing mild to moderate acne.
- Some medications can make acne worse; if so, he should discuss this with his doctor.
- Overenthusiastic cleaning can dry the skin, making it too sensitive for the use of topical treatments that might otherwise help, so get him to cleanse gently, using a mild fragrance free soap and water.
- He should apply acne medications over the entire affected area, not just on individual blemishes.

Eczema

Eczema affects about one in 12 adults, and occurs more frequently in men than in women. As there are different kinds of eczema, the causes depend on which type you have. **Atopic eczema** is thought to be hereditary, and may start as an allergic reaction to food or house dust. **Contact eczema** occurs when you come into direct contact with an irritant, such as chemicals, soaps, detergents, rubber, nickel or cement. **Seborrhoeic eczema** is thought to be caused by an overgrowth of yeast.

His doctor can prescribe emollients, which help reduce dryness and itching; topical steroids as a short-term measure to the skin to reduce inflammation; antibiotics; or anti-fungal creams for seborrhoeic eczema.

What you can do

- Traditional Chinese medicine (TCM) has a reputation for helping skin problems such as eczema but choose a reputable practitioner (see 'Useful addresses').
- Wool and synthetic fibres can irritate inflamed skin, so encourage him to wear cotton and other natural fibres.
- Overheating dries skin, leading to further irritation, so turn down the central heating and keep windows slightly open for at least some of the day.
- If eczema is severe, it is worth keeping a diary of chemicals he comes into contact with to see if anything triggers it. Common irritants are washing up liquid and washing powder.
- If he has atopic eczema, get rid of house dust mites as far as possible. Remove heavy carpets and curtains, vacuum carpets and mattresses thoroughly, and wash bedding frequently at high temperatures.
- Stress can worsen eczema so encourage him to learn a relaxation technique if possible, or go for a walk or swim or take some other form of non-competitive exercise.
- Atopic eczema is often allergy-related and may be helped by changing diet. Foods commonly found to worsen eczema include dairy, sugar, spicy foods, tea and coffee.
- Evening primrose oil has helped some people, either as a supplement or a cream.
- Try aromatherapy oils such as camomile, geranium, lavender and lemon balm.
- He could try taking a vitamin B complex supplement daily and

increasing his intake of vitamin A (found in liver, eggs, butter, milk and red and orange vegetables).
- A traditional home remedy is to rub a little cold-pressed olive oil into the affected area as it is rich in vitamin E.

Psoriasis

This is an immunological disease in which new skin cells reproduce too fast and rise to the skin surface before the dead ones have had time to be shed. The signs are patches of inflamed, red skin often with silvery scales on the scalp and hairline, the knees and elbows, and the small of the back. It can range in severity from the occasional mild patch to plaques covering a wide area of the body. Men and women are affected equally.

Experts are uncertain exactly why psoriasis develops. There is probably a genetic link, but it still seems to require a trigger. Common triggers include stress, infections like throat infections, medications like beta-blockers, or NSAIDs (non-steroidal anti-inflammatory drugs). Psoriasis tends to worsen during the winter, possibly because there is less sunlight and partly due to increased skin dryness caused by the cold weather and central heating.

He should see a doctor even if it is a mild attack as, left untreated, psoriasis can become severe and require hospital treatment, or cause complications such as psoriatic arthritis. His GP can prescribe emollient creams such as vitamin D creams, lotions, ointments and shampoos to help control the condition.

What you can do
- Coal tar is one of the oldest treatments and still effective, though some of the formulations are strong smelling and messy to use, and can stain the skin and clothing.
- As with acne, sunlight may be useful; or ultraviolet light therapy (phototherapy) is used in severe cases as it helps slow the overgrowth of the skin and reduce inflammation.
- A traditional remedy is to take at least one tablespoonful of cold-pressed olive oil a day, along with at least one raw vegetable salad. Rich in vitamin E, olive oil is emollient and can be used externally – just dab a little on the affected area.

- Liquorice root is another traditional herbal remedy for psoriasis. Use half a teaspoon of the powdered root in one cup of boiling water; sweeten with honey, allow to cool, and take three cups daily. (Large doses of liquorice can be laxative; it can also cause water retention and raised blood pressure and should not be taken if he has high blood pressure.)
- Or try nettle skin cream, or nettle tea made by infusing nettle tops in boiling water for ten minutes, then straining.
- He could try getting more vitamins A, C, E, B-complex; along with the mineral selenium.
- Also try and ensure he has enough protein in his diet.
- Psoriasis may be related to food intolerance, so see if it helps to exclude common allergens such as wheat and dairy produce from his diet for a while.
- Encourage him to cut down on sources of stress as some men find their condition becomes worse under stress.

Rosacea

Rosacea is an inflammatory skin condition that causes reddening or spiderveins of the face and occasionally of the trunk and limbs. The redness may be accompanied by spots or pustules that resemble acne – which is why rosacea is often mistakenly called adult acne. You do not develop whiteheads or blackheads.

Severe or untreated rosacea can cause tissue overgrowth on the nose, known as rhinophyma, more frequently in men than in women. It is also more common in fair-skinned people, although the exact cause is unknown.

What you can do

- Although it frequently clears up on its own, it is important to see your doctor as, apart from anything else, 25 per cent of people with rosacea develop eye complications which can range from mild to severe, with scarring of the eye and impaired vision. Treatment may consist of oral or topical antibiotics.
- It may also be worth looking for anything which triggers flushing such as alcohol, hot foods or drinks, spicy foods, or central heating.

Good skincare

Generally, and even if he does not have any of the above problems, there is plenty that can be done to promote good overall skin health:

- Encourage him to eat plenty of fresh fruit and vegetables.
- Drinking plenty of water (eight glasses a day) helps cleanse the system and keep skin hydrated.
- Smoking leads to premature wrinkling – yet another good excuse to stop.
- Wash regularly with mild, fragrance-free soap and rinse thoroughly – do not cleanse too enthusiastically as it can remove surface oils and lead to dryness and irritation.
- Do not soak in hot baths as this too is drying.
- Use a skin cream or moisturizer.
- Drying carefully between fingers and toes prevents irritation, cracking and other skin complications.
- He should wear protective gloves for DIY and gardening, and of course fully comply with any protective clothing issued at work against any substances likely to irritate the skin.

Those embarrassing problems

Bad breath

He may not thank you at first for drawing his attention to any bad breath and body odour, but with some men, sadly, unless you do, the problem may not go away. Morning breath is a practically universal condition in which the breath does not smell fresh because the flow of saliva has not yet been activated by taking in the day's food and drink. Garlic, smoking and alcohol can all cause the breath to smell, but the most common cause of bad breath is poor oral hygiene.

He can:

- clean his teeth at least twice a day, preferably after meals
- change his toothbrush every three months
- ensure dentures are kept scrupulously clean
- drink enough water to keep the flow of saliva going and his mouth hydrated, and chew sugar-free gum or eat fresh vegetables or fruit between meals
- visit his dentist regularly and if necessary consult him or her about the best method of brushing teeth
- consult his dentist about persistent bad breath as it may be due to gum infection. If the dentist does not find anything, consult your GP as bad breath can sometimes be a sign of underlying illness such as throat, lung or sinus infections, diabetes, kidney or liver disease
- try chewing on coriander seeds, cloves, cinnamon bark or some cardamon seeds, traditional remedies for bad breath
- chew on herbs such as parsley, rosemary, mint, tarragon and watercress
- drink fresh carrot, celery, watercress and cucumber juice with paprika – a traditional folk remedy
- try a mouthwash of water with a drop of the aromatherapy oils myrrh, thyme oil or fennel oil
- try acidophilus, found in live yoghurt, which may help with bad breath caused by incompletely digested food.

Body odour

The body has around two million sweat glands and produces more than three litres of sweat a day, most of which evaporates quickly without causing problems. Garlic, onions, curry or other spicy foods can cause body odour, as does stale sweat.

He should:

- change underwear and shower or bathe once a day
- be sure to dry himself properly to prevent bacteria living on moist skin (talc may help)
- wear loose natural fibres such as cotton and linen
- perhaps eat less meat as meat-eaters smell differently from vegetarians

- try yoga as some yoga postures are believed to lessen body and breath odour.

Footcare

It is easy for men to overlook feet and just put up with dead skin, corns or relatively minor conditions such as athlete's foot. However, feet are one of those areas where hygiene and health overlap, as neglected feet become increasingly uncomfortable and can even threaten the amount of physical activity taken.

Feet do need active care, not just regular passive soaks in the bath. As well as being thoroughly washed with soap, the dead skin also needs to be removed with a pumice stone, and toenails kept short and clean, as these are areas where infection such as athlete's foot can build up.

Worn-down or ill-fitting shoes should be thrown away, and socks in natural materials such as cotton worn to reduce sweating, perhaps with insoles of activated charcoal.

Try treating any corns and calluses with lemon juice as the citric acid helps to soften the skin (or try cider vinegar). Another natural remedy is crushed fresh garlic. For severe, persistent corns, calluses or bunions, see a chiropodist.

Athlete's foot, or tinea pedis, is sore, itchy skin between the toes, especially between the fourth and fifth toes, and is caused by a fungal infection. It tends to occur in people whose feet sweat a lot, for example if they play sport for a long time, as the moist heat generates the growth of fungal and yeast cells. Highly infectious, it can spread in changing rooms such as at public swimming pools. Good hygiene and footcare, however, go a long way towards preventing what can be a rather persistent condition once acquired. He should:

- treat with a powder that helps keep the area dry or with anti-fungal creams. Make sure you continue treating the skin for a couple of weeks after visible signs of the infection have gone as the infection can linger deep into the skin
- try putting a little live yoghurt on the affected area every day for its anti-fungal properties
- try a foot bath with aromatherapy oils such as tea tree and myrrh.

Both are good oils for skin problems as they have mild anti-fungal and anti-inflammatory properties

- treat shoes as they may be infected – old, smelly shoes should be thrown away
- wash feet thoroughly at least once a day. Soap feet and get rid of dead skin with a pumice stone
- wash feet after sports activities or physical work
- make sure the feet are thoroughly dried, especially between the toes
- use deodorant, anti-fungal preparations regularly on feet and shoes to prevent infection
- clean beneath the ends of the toenail, as a build-up of dead skin in this area forms the ideal breeding place for fungus.

7

Sexual health

In an ideal world, this area of health even more than others would look after itself effortlessly. However, sexual difficulties and impotence are surprisingly common, affecting at least one in five men. They may occur alone, or as part of an underlying physical condition such as heart trouble or diabetes, so that, even if he feels embarrassed or ashamed, checking them out with his doctor can be life-saving. Even if no cause can be found, much can be done to improve this area of health, and to treat any difficulties. Sexual fulfilment, while not necessary to all relationships, can make a significant contribution to good overall health.

What constitutes normal intimacy?

It is impossible to say! The sex drive varies so much from individual to individual, that even sex therapists cannot always define 'normal'. In men, the sex drive is affected by a range of hormones governed by the pituitary gland which stimulates the release of, among others, the male sex hormone testosterone.

Many factors can affect the production of these hormones, and sex drive varies from situation to situation. For example, desire which was strong on holiday or in the early part of a relationship may dwindle if he is working to a deadline on a demanding work project, or if there is a new baby. Money worries, the stress of a sick elderly parent, too much alcohol, can all affect desire. In fact, lack of desire affects an estimated 15 per cent of men at any one time.

It is certainly important not to feel that either of you 'should' be feeling a certain amount of desire, or that you 'should' be having sex a certain number of times a week or month. The important thing is that you both feel happy with the amount of intimacy you have, although problems should not be ignored.

71

Male erectile dysfunction

Erectile dysfunction (ED), or impotence, affects an estimated 10 per cent of men and relates to a more persistent inability to enjoy sex (as opposed to occasional loss of interest, as described above). While being a common source of jokes, it should always be taken seriously. Most doctors agree that, while some sexual dysfunction may be 'in the head', in many cases it can indicate an underlying medical condition.

Psychological causes

Sexual dysfunction can itself cause psychological problems such as anxiety, stress and depression. The main underlying psychological causes of dysfunction, however, can include:

- relationship problems
- sexual boredom
- stress and anxiety
- depression – 90 per cent of men with depression also have problems with impotence.

How can you tell if his impotence has a psychological cause? A clue may be whether his loss of interest in sex depends on conditions – for example, if desire returns after a good night's sleep, or on holiday, or at weekends when he is rested. If sex is possible under some circumstances or not others, then psychological reasons are more likely to be the cause of impotence. Simple self-help measures (see below) can also boost libido. If low libido persists in all circumstances, however, it is worth being medically checked to exclude the possibility of more serious conditions.

Physical causes

A range of physical conditions can affect sex drive and performance, including:

- Diabetes, the most common cause of sexual dysfunction. Erectile dysfunction affects 50–60 per cent of diabetic men.
- Heart trouble. Atherosclerosis, when the arteries become clogged

with fatty deposits, can result in inadequate blood flow to the penis. This causes about 40 per cent of erectile dysfunction in men over 50.

- Other conditions include high blood pressure, multiple sclerosis, kidney disease, fibrosis, hormonal imbalances, nerve damage and epilepsy and other neurological problems.
- Smoking cigarettes is implicated in up to 80 per cent of cases of erectile dysfunction, as it narrows the blood vessels and is a major cause of damage to the arteries leading to the penis. Men with high blood pressure who smoke are 26 times more likely to suffer erectile dysfunction.
- Too much alcohol, which can damage the nerves leading to the penis, reduce testosterone levels and increase levels of the female hormone oestrogen.
- Infection such as herpes or urethritis which may cause irritation or pain.
- The side effects of some prescribed drugs, particularly those used to treat high blood pressure, heart disease, depression, peptic ulcers and cancer.
- Age – nearly 20 per cent of men in their fifties have trouble compared with 7 per cent of those in their twenties.
- Structural problems. Rarely, men may be affected by problems such as Peyronie's disease (see below, 'Penile disorders').
- Low testosterone, involving symptoms such as exhaustion, irritability, loss of facial or body hair, shrinking testicles or muscle weakness.

Impotence – what you can do

- Do persuade him to see his GP, as any underlying causes need to be found and treated. In one study of 50 men who sought medical help for erectile dysfunction, although none of them had any obvious symptoms of heart disease, closer examination showed that they in fact had narrowed and blocked arteries, with 40 per cent of them at significant risk of angina or a heart attack.
- Get him to stop smoking (see Chapter 9, 'Other lifestyle factors', on how to help him give up). Just two cigarettes smoked before

sex markedly decrease blood flow to the penis and nicotine has a dose-related effect – the more he smokes, the less likely he is to manage sex.

- See if a period without alcohol helps him. After the first four to five units, alcohol stops being a stimulant and becomes a depressant, affecting the heart and respiratory system and lessening the ability to perform. Alcohol is thought to cause at least one in six cases of erectile dysfunction. Too much alcohol can result in fatty liver degeneration, which in turn can cause levels of testosterone to fall, so leading to drops in sex drive and sperm count.
- Regular aerobic exercise may help in many ways. It is very good for his heart and circulation, which play a major part in sexual performance. It also combats stress, which lowers libido and sex hormones, and obesity, which can also cause performance problems. Exercise can also boost physical confidence – important if he feels vulnerable because of any sexual difficulties. Allow two to three weeks for the benefits to be fully felt – encourage him to keep going!
- If he has diabetes, ensure it is properly controlled.
- Too much stress sends the adrenaline soaring so he cannot relax enough to make love. See Chapter 8, 'Work and stress', for suggestions on dealing with this. Rose oil is said to increase sperm count and quality and may act as a mild aphrodisiac. Add a few drops to his bath or blend with a light carrier oil such as almond for a soothing massage. If he is tense and anxious, the oil ylang ylang is relaxing.
- Likewise, try and ensure he gets enough sleep (see Chapter 9, 'Other lifestyle factors').

Nutrients

Zinc deficiency is believed to be behind some male impotence and infertility. Zinc is essential for sperm formation and health, and men who have zinc deficiencies may produce zero, or reduced, sperm counts. This mineral also helps regulate testosterone, and zinc deficiency before adolescence can result in smaller male sex organs and low libido. Stress, caffeine, smoking and alcohol all increase the need for zinc. Good sources of zinc are oysters, other seafood, red meat, wholegrains, pulses, eggs, cheese, peanuts, sunflower seeds, oatmeal, yeast and milk.

Vitamin E has been tested as a supplement for subfertility and the quality of sperm is related to the amount of vitamin E in a man's diet. Vitamin E protects the sex hormones from destruction by oxygen, strengthens muscle fibres and helps absorb free radicals. Good sources include vegetables, margarine, eggs, butter and wheatgerm.

Watercress leaves are a traditional home remedy and are supposed to act as a sexual tonic; so are sesame and pumpkin seeds, which are rich in essential fatty acids. Generally, keep your diet low in fat to reduce the risk of atherosclerosis; ensure he is eating enough protein as a lack of it can cause libido to fall and sperm count to lessen; include lots of coloured vegetables such as green, red and yellow peppers, broccoli and spinach, all of which contain antioxidants which absorb free radicals and reduce the risk of heart disease, a common source of impotence in men.

Herbs

The following herbs have ancient reputations for balancing or toning sexual energies. You should consult your doctor if you are suffering a medical condition or are taking any medication before trying them, and you should not exceed any recommended dose:

- **agnus castus:** *vitex agnus-castus* is supposed to work by correcting hormonal imbalances and balancing sexual energy.
- **damiana:** *turnera aphrodisiaca* has long been used as an aphrodisiac and tonic, especially among the Mexican Indians. It is believed to contain alkaloids which help raise levels of testosterone.
- **saw palmetto:** *serenoa serrulata* is supposed to act directly on the sex hormones. It contains the active constituents steroidal saponins, structurally similar to human sex hormones. However, while it seems to promote prostate health (see Chapter 3), one American study found that the herb did not live up to its anecdotal reputation for improving sex. (If you plan to try it, do not take it if you are pregnant.) A doctor should be consulted for all prostate problems.

75

- **yohimbe:** from the African tree *corynanthe yohimbe or pausinys-talis yohimbe*, this is widely viewed as the most effective natural aphrodisiac. Yohimbe bark contains yohimbine, an alkaloid said to help blood flow to the pelvic area and erectile tissues. Some clinical trials have shown that yohimbe can increase blood flow to the penis. Do not take if you have high blood pressure and consult your doctor before taking it if you have any heart condition.

Talking about it

Robert would make various excuses not to have sex – he was too tired, he was worried he had an infection on his penis, he wanted to be fresh for the next day's work, he did not want to make love to her while she was pregnant, he was afraid the children would come in, and so on. His partner Marie was feeling increasingly hurt and began to wonder if he was having an affair – in fact, after this situation persisted for several months, she began to feel like having an affair herself.

Both impotence and infertility can drive a rift between couples, so keeping the channels of communication open is important. He may be feeling guilty and ashamed, worrying that his masculinity is threatened, or blaming himself – or you. You in turn may be feeling rejected and confused, especially if, as often happens, he refuses to confide in you or to discuss his health worries.

Talk to your partner, encourage him to be open, and bear in mind that intimacy is not confined to sex. Try and stay physically close to your partner by cuddling or sharing the same bed, as it helps keep you emotionally close.

This is a time when you need both to give and receive support, so talk to friends you trust, too, or a fertility counsellor. He may also benefit from talking to other men in the same situation (see 'Useful addresses' for support organizations).

Treatment

Viagra (sildenafil) is still probably the best-known treatment for impotence, although it is not an aphrodisiac and has no effect unless the person is sexually stimulated. It works by helping to relax the blood vessels in the penis, so promoting better blood flow. The most common side effects are headaches and facial flushing, and it cannot be taken by men who are also using medicines containing nitrates (commonly prescribed for angina).

Hormonal treatments may also be used in the relatively few cases where low testosterone is the cause of erectile dysfunction. Your doctor should measure your testosterone level first to confirm that it really is low.

Otherwise, the range of rather cumbersome local therapies for erectile dysfunction goes some way towards explaining the initial enthusiasm for Viagra. Injection therapy is when the penis is injected with a drug which relaxes the blood vessels and muscles, allowing increased blood flow. MUSE (medicated urethral system for erection) is when a small pellet containing a drug is inserted into the urethra via a plastic device. Vacuum therapy involves fitting a cylindrical device round the penis, pumping the air out until the penis fills with blood. Once it has become hard enough, a plastic constricting ring is placed around the base of the penis to trap the blood. All militate against spontaneity as well as sometimes causing discomfort and bruising.

Complications of injection therapy may include fibrosis (scar tissue in the penis), or, more serious, priapism, or prolonged erection, a medical emergency which can destroy the ability to have an erection for good (see below, 'Penile disorders').

Surgical implants, which tend to be used as a last resort, involve inserting devices within the penis which help keep it rigid. Again, this may not be as firm as a natural erection and may also involve complications in terms of infection or failure of the implant.

Given the generally poor state of men's health today, it may be better to try improving his general well-being before trying these therapies out – although they can and do work successfully for many. However, they do only work on the penis – they do not tackle obesity, poor diet, lack of exercise, anxiety, or any of the other ills modern man is so prone to!

Sex therapy

Some people may benefit from psychosexual counselling. Apart from helping with difficulties which have a psychological cause, it can also provide helpful support when used in combination with other treatment, and may sometimes be needed after any physical problems have been sorted out.

Robert had had problems for two years due to poorly controlled diabetes, and his self-esteem had plummeted. He needed a lot of reassurance from Marie, and a few sessions with a sexual therapist, before he could come to terms with what had happened and regain his sexual confidence.

Therapy may also help you as a couple, if you are trying to re-establish intimacy after a period of enforced abstinence, or if you need to address underlying emotions which have caused sexual difficulties apart from his impotence.

Infertility

Like impotence, infertility is common, affecting around one in six couples, and a major cause is the male inability to produce enough healthy sperm. Generally, the number of sperm has almost halved in recent years, with a large increase in the numbers of abnormal sperm. Increasing pollution is thought to be a factor. Long hours of driving do not help as they warm the testicles which produce more sperm when cooler. However, becoming pregnant does take time even with the most fertile couples – around a year is considered normal.

Reasons for infertility include:

- sperm problems which may affect normal shaping and/or motility (the ability to move into the fallopian tube where the egg is fertilized). Sperm problems can be caused by a wide range of conditions including reduced sperm as an after-effect of mumps, trapped sperm inside the testicles, sexually transmitted infections, testicles that were undescended at birth, genetic reasons, enlarged veins round the testicles (varicoceles), and, rarely, hormonal causes;

- ejaculation problems, for example retrograde or 'dry' ejaculation;
- disorders such as diabetes may affect the nervous system so that semen cannot be pumped into the urethra;
- erectile dysfunction (impotence).

A wide range of treatments exist, not just to help fertility but also for any underlying physical conditions which could affect fertility – for example, antibiotics for infections, surgery to remove varicoceles or blockages in the testicles, or medication for some ejaculation problems, e.g. to tighten the bladder neck in cases of retrograde ejaculation.

Treatments for fertility itself include hormonal treatments, such as clomiphene, for a low sperm count with no obvious explanation, assisted conception techniques such as IUI (intrauterine insemination), when sperm are selected and then placed in your womb. IVF (in vitro fertilization) and ICSI (intra-cytoplasmic sperm injection) are also options. Donor insemination using another man's sperm is another possibility.

What you can do

Simple changes may be enough to tip the balance in cases of subfertility, but do not delay in asking for help. Fertility investigations and treatment take time – and many couples find that while they are waiting, pregnancy occurs naturally.

- Check whether any medication he is taking could be affecting his sperm quality, such as anabolic steroids, some blood pressure drugs, and some anti-depressants, and ask your GP about alternatives.
- He should also visit his GP if he has had problems in the past such as undescended testicles, mumps, or surgery in the pelvic area to repair a hernia. As well as taking a medical history to find out if any past or present condition could have affected his fertility, your

GP can arrange for tests such as semen analysis and sperm function tests and genetic tests.

- Ask your GP to test for infection as well so he or she can prescribe antibiotics to treat any underlying infection. Vitamin E supplements may improve sperm quality in some men who have high quantities of free radicals as a result of subclinical or unrealized infections.
- He should also check out any worrying symptoms connected with sex, such as pain on ejaculation, erection problems, low volume of semen, blood in the semen and so on.
- You should also make an appointment to assess your fertility.
- A cannabis joint may be relaxing, but can affect sperm manufacture for 36 hours.
- Many vaginal lubricants kill sperm, so avoid them if you are trying to become pregnant.
- Abstaining from ejaculation seven to ten days before your ovulation can improve chances of conception as it increases sperm count. Ovulation, during which you are fertile, is usually between 12 to 19 days before your next period and may be characterized by increased vaginal secretions, increased desire, and a distinctive, sharpish pain which may continue for a day in the left or right ovary (a few inches in from the top of the pelvis) caused by the egg bursting.
- Heat affects sperm formation, so suggest he avoids hot baths, wears loose underwear (cotton boxer shorts) and bathes the testicles with cold water regularly.
- He can also give up alcohol for a while – 40 per cent of subfertility in men is linked with drinking just four units of alcohol a day.
- Suggest that he reduces caffeine intake to no more than three cups of tea, coffee or cola a day.
- Among its other evils, smoking causes free radicals which affect sperm quality.
- He should lose any excess weight, as it can create hormonal imbalances involving testosterone and oestrogen which affect fertility.
- Foods that contain essential fatty acids (EFAs) are believed to stimulate the production of sex hormones. They include oily fish,

fish liver oils, seeds, nuts, pulses, beans, evening primrose oil and unrefined vegetable oils. His fertility may benefit from supplements of vitamin C, betacarotene and zinc.

- Low levels of zinc have been associated with male infertility – see above, 'Herbs and nutrients'. Lack of vitamin B6 has also been linked with low sperm count. This is best taken as part of a vitamin B complex or via food sources including meat, fish, milk, eggs, wholegrain cereals and vegetables.
- Some herbs, especially in high concentrations, may affect sperm motility and should be avoided if couples are having fertility problems, according to some American research. The herbs include St John's wort, echinacea, ginkgo biloba and saw palmetto.
- Certain complementary remedies appear to have helped some people with fertility problems. Several studies (from China, Japan and Germany) have shown that acupuncture can help male and female infertility, and may improve the quantity and quality of sperm. Traditional Chinese medicine is also helpful, according to other research.

> Lawrence was relatively young – just 31 – but he and his partner Rosie had been trying for a baby for three years, and had been undergoing infertility treatment for the last 14 months. Her patience was running out and she decided she wanted IVF and a baby right now! Lawrence wanted them both to try complementary remedies first, but while she agreed to try a healthier lifestyle (cutting out alcohol, eating properly and so on) she felt that 'time was running out'. However, he tried a course of acupuncture while she was waiting for IVF, and persuaded her to have a go too. Four months later she conceived. Neither was quite sure whether the acupuncture had helped – but they tried it again when wanting to conceive a second child, and again Rosie became pregnant after a few months of treatment.

Penile disorders

Your partner should seek medical advice if he is at all concerned about any symptoms of penile disorder.

Peyronie's disease, which is believed to affect some 80,000 men in the UK, is a condition in which the penis becomes curved during an erection. There may be benign lumps (plaques) in the penile tissue which cause thickening and sometimes pain on erection. The cause is unknown but may be due to minor penile damage which causes internal bleeding. Mild cases usually heal within a few months; more severe cases may be treated by surgery. Vitamin E supplements may help in some cases.

Hypospadias is when the opening of the urethra is not at its normal place at the end of the penis and may also cause the penis to bend. It affects about one in every 300 males and usually runs in families, although the exact cause is unknown. Severe hypospadias is usually noticed at birth and corrected by operation in infancy. Uncorrected or slight hypospadias can still be corrected by surgery as an adult.

Balanitis is inflammation of the head of the penis with red patches, soreness and itchiness. Common in uncircumcised men, it is usually associated with poor hygiene, and can be prevented by washing under the foreskin. Severe balanitis may be a sign of diabetes, so you should see your doctor – also to make sure it has not been caused by a sexually transmitted infection which produces similar symptoms.

Paraphimosis is a painful condition in which the foreskin cannot be pulled back over the head of the penis. This may be the result of infection, poor personal hygiene, or damage to the penis, causing swelling. Good hygiene helps prevent it but see your doctor in case treatment is needed for infection.

Phimosis is an unusually tight foreskin that cannot be drawn back from the head of the penis and again merits a visit to the doctor.

Priapism, a medical emergency, is a prolonged erection (for more than four hours) that, if left untreated, can permanently damage the penis. In most cases the cause is unknown, although it can sometimes be a side effect of certain drugs. This is a medical emergency as it can lead to permanent impotence if left untreated because of the risk of clotting as the blood fails to drain out of the penis. Priapism merits a visit to the nearest accident and emergency unit, although ice packs or movement might relieve some of the pain.

8
Work and stress

The type of work a man does not only has an impact on his health, but may even be linked with his lifespan. For example, unskilled men have a higher death rate than do professional men in many diseases, such as CHD. The premature death rate from CHD for male manual workers, such as builders and cleaners, is 58 per cent higher than for male non-manual workers, such as doctors and lawyers. According to death statistics compiled by the Registrar General, the death rate for executives is as good as for lawyers and much better than for skilled workers – who are in turn better than unskilled. But, in turn, executives are not as long-lived as are clergymen or higher civil servants. There is also a geographical factor, with better health in men who work in the south and east of the UK, and poorer health in those who work in the north and west.

Executive health

Certain problems may plague high fliers in particular – stress, frustration, irregular time schedules, travel fatigue and jet lag, possible health problems abroad, a poor or irregular diet. All can play havoc with an executive's health, causing digestive problems, sleep problems and irritability as just initial symptoms of the disturbance to health. These can and do progress to more serious conditions such as high blood pressure and coronary heart disease.

Executive stress is a cliché, yet too many hardworking men do nothing to tackle it. To a certain extent, executives may have less stress than subordinates as they may be more in control of their time and activities, and have more power. It depends on how urgent their internal stressors are – such as the pressure to do a good job, to achieve more and more, to meet certain standards, and so on.

Symptoms of stress at work may include:

- loss of self-confidence
- loss of confidence in those under him

83

- taking on too much power and responsibility, and delegating less
- tendency to ask for more and more information before making a decision, and difficulty in making decisions
- overactivity but less in the way of results (running round in circles) or being scattered and unfocused
- turning down holidays
- repeated short sickness leave
- self-pity and irritability
- talking too much
- drinking too much
- doing more and more activities at home instead of relaxing.

See the end of this chapter on how to deal with stress.

Sleep problems, including insomnia, can be among the most troublesome complaints of executives.

Gordon, a professor of economics, would wake repeatedly during the night, or early in the morning, finding his night left him unrefreshed. Like many other hard workers, he also had trouble falling asleep, and problems and situations from the day would go round and round his head. A strong nightcap or two 'to relax' was the obvious solution – posing further threats to his health.

Jan, a high-ranking executive in a musical company, would fall asleep easily, but wake between 2 a.m. and 5 a.m. worrying about the day ahead.

For suggestions on dealing with sleep problems, see Chapter 9 on 'Other lifestyle factors'. Bear in mind that regular early morning waking, a classic symptom of depression and anxiety, may also herald physical illness, so it is worth checking out at the doctor's as well.

Travel

The design and situation of airports, and all the hanging around entailed, are trying enough. With increased fears of terrorism and extra security, flying has become even more stressful. Jetlag is also a reality for many frequent fliers.

What you can do

- Suggest he learn some meditation technique to practise while waiting for flights, taxis and so on.
- Light meals are best while travelling. Drinking plenty of water before, during and after flying prevents dehydration.
- He can ask his doctor for a sedative to take just while travelling, although it may be better to explore herbal soothers first such as balm, lavender, chamomile, passiflora. Ginseng may also help.
- He can try and walk about while waiting to board, and during long haul flights.
- Changing time zones can slow thinking down, so if possible he should try and leave himself a day or a few hours at least after arrival, and not plunge straight into meetings. Melatonin has been recommended for jetlag.
- He should check whether immunization is needed for distant parts of the world.
- Travellers' diarrhoea can be an occupational hazard. While abroad, he should avoid fruit salads, cold meats and ice, and go for freshly cooked foods, and bottled water.
- A reminder about sun safety may not come amiss if he travels to hot climes – not too much exposure and, in the event of sunstroke or heatstroke, rest and lots of drinks.

Commuting

Travel fatigue is a fact of life for many who spend time commuting – an hour or more in the car or on a train is in itself stressful, never mind the work as well. While maybe just one accident in a thousand is due to illness while driving, travel stress can tax the heart and make it work harder. Drivers are well-documented as suffering an increased heart rate in heavy traffic, poor driving conditions, and after a near miss.

Sources of stress for commuters are manifold – overcrowding, overheating or lack of heat, late services, cancellations, and security alerts. Uncertainty about transport can have a knock-on effect on other areas of life, and may involve lifestyle changes such as having to make an earlier start, getting less sleep, and anxiety about being on time. Prolonged over a period of time, this too can lead to illness.

What you can do

- If he drives, suggest he stops for a break at least once every two hours.
- Buy him some soothing cassettes for the car – music, natural sounds, or positive affirmations.
- He should leave his mobile switched off while driving – research shows that people talking on mobiles while driving have slower reaction times than those who have been drinking.
- Perhaps he could discuss flexi-time with his boss so that he comes in early and leaves early to avoid the rush hour. Another option to negotiate is working more from home. Moving house or changing jobs may be the only solution for some.

> Paul commuted an hour and three-quarters to work via train and tube and after three years felt his health was suffering. He wanted to move nearer but his partner was reluctant to uproot herself and their two children from an area where they were settled with friends and schools. Paul compromised and took a less well-paid job 15 minutes' drive away – his partner felt that a drop in salary was a good exchange for the fact that he now saw much more of her and the children.

Health and safety at work

Nine out of ten fatal accidents at work involve men. Boredom and tiredness are the biggest factors in industrial accidents, and most accidents occur in the afternoons or early evening. Enough sleep, getting fit and regular breaks can all help prevent accidents, as can increased safety awareness, and as many changes in routine (both at home and at work) as he can implement.

One major health risk in the UK is RSI (repetitive strain injury) of which there are an estimated 100,000 new cases a year – with a working population of 26 million, maybe more. A keyboard is the main risk factor. He can prevent this by having a proper work station, taking breaks, and not making it worse – for example, by hunching the phone under his neck and typing during a phone call. He should also inform his employer and health and safety department.

Stress

Stress is the spice of life, boosting energy, coping and reaction skills, but like spice needs to be used in moderation. We all need change – a house move, a new friend, a new job, and the feeling of not knowing what will happen next is great – so long as we feel we have some measure of control, even if it is just by being in charge of our own reactions to events.

When we talk of stress, we usually mean too much stress relating to events where we feel powerless. Around 60 per cent of all absences from work (some 40 million working days a year) are thought to be related to this kind of stress. Physical symptoms include headaches, backache, dry mouth, indigestion, sexual problems and sleep problems. Common mental symptoms include poor concentration and organization, memory problems, feelings of isolation and frustration, irritability and anger, depression and panic attacks.

Stress tends to have a negative escalating effect in that the longer it is left to go on untackled, the worse it tends to get, often causing a range of negative feelings and behaviour and affecting the way a person copes at home and work. Stress affects the whole body, lowering immunity and increasing the risk of disease. For example, there is good evidence that stress increases susceptibility to a wide range of illnesses, from the common cold to cancer.

Stress may also worsen a range of conditions, such as skin conditions such as psoriasis and eczema, irritable bowel syndrome, diabetes, asthma, epilepsy, heart disease, high blood pressure, hair loss and sexual problems.

Derek was everyone's friend and a champion of everyone's cause but the word 'no' was not in his vocabulary and he was burning out. His wife Annie could see the danger signs – he was irritable, disorganized, increasingly less effective with his time, and feeling very put upon. She was always reminding him that charity began at home and that he could not save the whole world. However, it was not until Derek broke his ankle and had to stay put for a while that he really realized that he had to let go of some of the people and activities in his life.

Bob would talk about how much his job as a web technician was stressing him but do nothing about it. He genuinely felt trapped by the limited options he could see around him and was nervous about leaving to start his own business, which he was fully equipped to do. His wife Marie was fast running out of sympathy – she was fed up of listening to him talk and do nothing, and could also see that he was suffering increasing physical symptoms of stress such as faintness and panic attacks.

So what do you do? Your power over another person – especially sometimes your nearest and dearest – is limited! But you can start by trying to find out whether it is really circumstances that are causing the upset, or whether it lies more within his personality – that is, whether the stressor is internal or external:

- internal stressors could be perfectionism; low self-esteem; not doing what you really want to in life; lack of direction or having unclear goals; fear of the unknown or of change; working long hours and being unable to pace yourself, slow down or relax and unwind; loneliness or boredom;
- external stressors could be bereavement, relationship breakdown, moving house, new job or loss of job, change in health, change in financial status, time constraints.

Of the two, external stressors are easier to manage as, with time and support from others, most situations can be changed – for example, the man who hates his job may eventually be able to find a new one. Conversely, internal stressors need changing from within – more challenging and difficult for some people, who repeatedly try and soothe internal stressors by changing external ones. The man who changes his job is not going to escape his workaholism unless he changes his attitude too.

To help him find out whether his stress is internal or external, you could try asking him the following questions:

- What is the stress really telling you?
- Is it a valid or useful feeling? For example, does it point out a gap between where you are now and where you want to be?
- What would you really like to be doing with your life?

- What is it that stops you getting there?
- What do you have to do to change it?

How to help

As Bob's story suggests, tackling the cause of the stress is the most effective way of dealing with it, whether it is tiresome commuting, an unsatisfactory job, or unreasonable family demands. Stress must be tackled, though – if it boils over into anger, this can be destructive to his health. Hostile, angry men run the risk of high blood pressure, whether their hostility is expressed or not.

- Help him work out which situations cause him stress and why. A stress diary might help, in which to note sources of stress, and how he reacted.
- Encourage him to take proper action, rather than just talking about it and indulging in behaviour that acts as a temporary soother such as smoking, comfort eating, and drinking too much. Instead, try and work out a step-by-step plan for dealing with the root cause of the stress.
- Discuss ways he could make his work environment more friendly. Stress can come from noise, an uncomfortable chair, or poor lighting, so see if he can negotiate any improvements.
- Insist that he delegate and not wearily take the world on his shoulders because 'no one else can do it right'.
- Encourage him to take plenty of regular exercise. Endurance exercise, such as walking, running, cycling, or swimming, is well-documented as a great stress reliever. A break at lunchtime, say for a walk or swim, may be especially helpful as it gets him away from any work pressures.
- Encourage him to avoid stressors such as alcohol and caffeine. Mix decaffeinated with caffeinated coffee, serve herbal teas.
- Being overweight can be stressful so arrange the daily diet so he does not have to struggle with tempting puddings, high fat food and so on.
- Try and arrange the bedroom to encourage adequate sleep most nights of the week (see section on sleep in Chapter 9).
- Some people have found complementary therapies and relaxation

techniques very helpful in combating stress, including acupressure, flotation therapy, homeopathy, hypnotherapy, meditation, massage and yoga.

- Setting the alarm 20 minutes earlier in the morning cuts down on stressful rushing.
- Encourage him to drive in a more leisurely way – again, leaving ten minutes earlier might help. The few minutes gained by aggressive driving is just not worth the stress.
- Keep communication gadgets under control such as email, mobile phones and faxes. Answerphones and voicemail are there for a reason. (See section on 'Communication' below.)
- Arrange breaks from the routine, such as day trips or dinners with friends. Many women find if they do not do this, it does not get done – yet the man really appreciates it when it has been arranged.
- Suggest he take a minute out when the stress is mounting. Teach him yoga deep breathing from the abdomen rather than the chest.
- Suggest he take some time for pursuits that are not essential or necessary. This could be leisure, voluntary work, something that is just for him, such as a walk or a sleep, or something that is for somebody else, like taking the kids to the park or helping a neighbour take rubbish to the tip.
- Encourage him to be as positive as possible – try and keep hostile gossip to a minimum, and accept and learn from past mistakes. Human error is part of life.
- Encourage him to mix with people, whether it is friends, a sports club, social activity or volunteer work. Seeing others takes the edge off personal stress and puts personal problems into perspective.
- Get him to see his doctor if you feel that his stress levels are not improving, or if he experiences worrying physical symptoms.

Communication

Poor communication is stressful, especially when it comes from work superiors. The arts of speaking your mind, and of listening, can be overlooked in surprisingly obvious ways.

Eric's boss (who worked in another town) insisted that all his communications take place by email – to save time and keep everything clear, he said. This made Eric's blood pressure rise as there were times when he needed a two-minute chat to clarify minor points, or when he needed an immediate answer. Eric knew his boss was under a great deal of pressure and that email was his way of keeping the stress at bay, but Eric felt he had been put in an impossible position, and that this mode of communication was adding to his own stress level in no small way.

In this case, the challenge was for Eric to improve his own communication skills so as to get through to his boss. Learning to say what he really thought was not easy. In the end he did pick up the phone to his boss and vented his frustration in the most tactful way he could. His boss was rather taken aback and said he had meant email to be a general rule not an unbreakable one. The verbal communication relieved everyone's stress.

Unfortunately, both verbal and non-verbal communication can be used in an aggressive way at work. Work rage or 'aggression' is on the rise, according to some experts, who blame increasing pressure on employees to do more and more, with growing insecurity about their jobs.

Work rage tends to be verbal rather than physical – for example, spreading false rumours or laughing at someone behind their back; interrupting the person; not returning their phone calls; ignoring them; arriving late for meetings; and so on. To a certain extent this behaviour is too commonplace to cause concern and often says more about the one who engages in it, than about the supposed victim. Taken as part of an ongoing pattern, however, it can be demoralizing. Your partner should inform his manager or superior, who should take immediate action, not make excuses for the aggressor, or look the other way.

Get organized

Few matters cause such frustration as never knowing where to find the car keys, and chronic disorganization can cause a lot of stress over time, perhaps by making him late for work on a regular basis and so setting the stage for more stress. It takes minimal effort to get organized with small changes, such as always putting keys in the same place like a hook in the hall, preparing work clothes and packed lunches the night before, and leaving the kitchen tidy so that breakfast is easier.

The same applies to clutter. Help him go through and throw out old, outworn clothes and shoes. Sort papers into labelled and dated boxes. Unless you need it for tax or work reference, throw papers away after a year.

Procrastination is another great stressor (and, like disorganization, may itself be a sign of stress).

Andrew had originally attracted Andrea because he was so laid back. Now, however, he was driving her mad because his way of dealing with bills was to put the unopened envelope in a drawer. Likewise, he would never get petrol until they seemed in danger of running out. She felt she was always picking up after him.

So, plan and act. Arrange for bills to be paid by direct debit or pay bills as soon as they come in; if you have difficulty paying, contact the company at once and see if you can arrange to defer or part-pay. Keep the petrol tank filled up to avoid the desperate stop at the garage when he is already late for work, and so on. Keeping on top of the daily minutiae makes for clearer heads all round.

Change is possible

If he is really stressed with work, or is worried about losing his job, dislikes it but sticks with it only for the money, you can help him explore ways out.

Help him research an alternative lifestyle. Together, write down a list of everything he can do, from putting up a shelf or cooking a good pilaff, to reading German or having a flair for crossword puzzles. Then look at the list to see if any of these could be used to earn money, and take some action, however small, to start creating a new reality.

Look at new skills he could learn. These could be allied to his job, or outside it. Two heads are often better than one, and once you start putting some energy into thinking creatively, new solutions may well appear. Do not let him suffer in silence because he feels there is no alternative.

9

Other lifestyle factors

As you must have gathered, one of the key points about men's health is that much of it is in their own hands – which often means, in your hands. Self-destructive and aggressive behaviours have been highlighted again and again as a directly contributing factor to the poor state of male health. If men really are becoming the new women, then hopefully in time they may learn 'female' survival skills, too! Meantime, whatever methods you can use to modify his lifestyle can only help.

Part of this is improving awareness – again, not just in your man, but in any children, encouraging sons to be responsible for themselves. Willingness to hear about preventative healthcare and lifestyle varies from man to man. A man who has just come home from the doctor with a diagnosis of high blood pressure may be a lot more willing to listen than the one who left the house for the surgery an hour before.

Accidents

Read any medical literature about men and you would think they spent their entire time having accidents. Accidents are the third biggest premature killer of men after heart disease and cancer and, among younger men under 35, road accidents are the biggest cause of death, accounting for 21 per cent of deaths in this age group. Young men (16–34) in particular are more than twice as likely than women to have accidents.

Men are much more often involved in accidents at work than are women, perhaps because the nature of their work is often more dangerous or because their behaviour or actions put them at greater risk. Women also tend to work part-time more, which in itself reduces risks. According to RoSPA (Royal Society for the Prevention of Accidents), the disparity between men and women in fatal accidents is even more marked – around 5,600 men and 330 women die in a year as a result of an accident at work. And, in the UK, there are still 1.6 million workplace injuries every year as well as 2.2 million cases of ill health caused, or made worse, by work.

According to RoSPA again, however, more people are injured in their own homes than anywhere else, with home accidents accounting for 37 per cent of all accidents requiring hospital treatment in a year. Falls account for nearly 40 per cent of all home accidents, while fire is another major preventable home hazard.

Discussing safety with your man can be a useful starting preventative strategy, to raise his awareness. Otherwise, there are a number of actions you can take.

Helping him reduce risks

- He should insist on appropriate health and safety measures at work if these are lacking.
- Look round the house for any obvious risks. Check for worn and loose-fitting carpets, poor lighting – especially on stairs – unguarded fires, cracked plugs and worn flexes, furniture too close to fires and so on.
- Discourage dangerous habits like dumping tools at the top of the cellar stairs. Ensure stairs and landing floors are always kept clear.
- Have appliances checked for safety and use them correctly.
- Install smoke alarms.
- Accidents are more likely to happen if he is tired, stressed or unwell. Other causes of accidents include impatience, carelessness, inadequate knowledge and training (for example when tackling electrical projects), alcohol, drugs and medicines. As far as possible, tactfully try and ensure he is fully equipped in every sense for any DIY jobs he takes on.
- Persuade him to drive more slowly and safely, avoid drinking and driving, and to always wear a seat belt.
- Suggest he has regular eye tests.
- Contact RoSPA for further information (see 'Useful addresses').

Alcohol

A couple of glasses of wine with dinner are taken for granted as one of life's rightful pleasures in many parts of Europe, where alcoholism rates are on the whole declining. In the UK, however, rates of alcoholism are rapidly increasing and once again the chief culprits are men, who insist on treating it as a drug rather than a tool of civilization. More than a quarter of all men drink too much, and 36 per cent drink excessively. One in eight admissions to hospital from casualty are alcohol-related and most are men, while more than a quarter of all hospital admissions are related to the effects of alcohol.

The bad effects of long-term alcohol abuse are well-known, although some are better known than others. For example, most people realize that alcohol can destroy the liver, but may not always realize that it also kills off brain cells. Too much alcohol over a period of time can cause memory loss, intellectual deterioration, depression and eventually dementia. It affects the heart, making high blood pressure, heart attacks and stroke more likely. It can also damage the digestive system, causing gastritis, pancreatitis, peptic ulcer and cancer of the mouth, throat or oesophagus. Nerves too may suffer, resulting in numbness, tingling and weakness, and also causing impotence and infertility. As far as the liver is concerned, there is a range of disorders which may result apart from cirrhosis, including fatty liver degeneration and liver cancer. Last but not least are the cosmetic changes – flushed skin, rheumy eyes, pot belly, bad breath and so on.

Warning signs

You can probably tell if your partner is drinking too much but it may not always be obvious to him, or, if he knows it deep down, he may not be willing to admit it.

- Drinking to change his mood – for example, he may drink to relieve depression or to escape from a bad day at work.
- He seems to feel uncomfortable on a day without a drink.
- Drink is affecting his life significantly, for example it makes him late for work or he cannot get out of bed on Saturday to go shopping or take the kids out.
- He seems to crave a drink.
- He is secretive or untruthful about his drinking.
- He obviously feels or says life is not worth living without alcohol – a statement which should make you prick up your ears and

96

probably take more drastic action (see below, 'Helping him cut down').

Helping him cut down

Just how frank should you be when trying to tackle your man's drinking? This can be an even more delicate question than other aspects of male health. First, you need to talk to him when he is sober – if the problem is that bad. It may just be a question of getting him to cut down a bit. But if you feel you are having to deal with a serious problem, get help. If his drinking is very bad and he will not listen to reason, or if he constantly breaks promises to stop, and your life is being affected, it is very important to get support for yourself, such as Al-Anon for the families and friends of alcoholics. At some point you may have to give up trying to change him, and attend to your own life and your own needs.

Men are advised to keep their average weekly intake of alcohol below 21 units. A unit of alcohol, roughly around eight grams, can be a half of beer, a glass of wine or sherry, or a single measure of spirits.

- If you are the one to buy wines and so on, look for lower-alcohol varieties and try serving them mixed with lots of lemonade, tonic water or other soft drinks to quench thirst.
- Encourage him to set a limit before starting to drink and to stick to it.
- Suggest he have 'days off' to give his liver a chance to recover.
- Point out that drink causes weight gain, bad breath and red, rheumy eyes!
- Keep a drink diary and show it to him after a few weeks – it may be an eye-opener for you both.
- Get him to contact the family doctor or to contact a support group such as Alcoholics Anonymous or Alcohol Concern. There is plenty of support online as well, such as Rational Recovery (see 'Useful addresses').

Smoking

Around 28 per cent of men still smoke and the average smoker gets through 111 cigarettes a week. The attractions of nicotine still outweigh its well-publicized health risks for many. These include the fact that, according to ASH (Action on Smoking and Health), several hundred people die every year from breathing others' cigarette smoke. Passive smoking is also linked with cot death and causes 4,000 miscarriages a year, as well as congenital defects, causing asthma, eczema and glue ear in young children. The children of men who smoke are twice as likely to develop leukaemia or cancer of the lymph nodes (lymphoma), more likely to develop any childhood cancer, and 40 per cent more likely to develop brain tumours than are the children of non-smoking fathers.

The results of smoking for the smoker are also stark: one in two smokers will die as a result of their habit. Smoking causes a third of all cancer deaths, including the majority of lung cancer deaths. It also causes four out of five deaths from bronchitis and emphysema, and one in four deaths from heart disease. No part of the body is unaffected. Two thousand arms and legs are amputated every year in the UK as a direct result of smoking.

The advantages of giving up smoking are also well-publicized and often broken down into hour-by-hour or even minute-by-minute gains to encourage those who find it hard to give up. For example, within 20 minutes blood pressure and pulse fall significantly; within eight hours the blood regains its normal oxygen level and poisonous carbon monoxide is excreted; within 24 hours the chance of a heart attack drops; and within 48 hours nerve endings start to grow and the senses of smell and taste start to become sharper.

In general terms, stopping smoking increases life expectancy especially if you give up before 30 – non-smokers live on average six years longer than smokers. It also boosts general fitness, health and well-being, including sexual performance (because of reduced blood flow, smoking can cause erectile dysfunction and affect the quality of sperm). It also leaves more money for other pursuits – a 20-a-day cigarette habit costs well over £1,000 a year.

Giving up is notoriously difficult but not, as some have suggested, impossible. It can be done, and has been done by thousands. All that is really needed is motivation.

Helping him give up

Only he can give up. However, there are a number of ways in which you may be able to help:

- If he has agreed to give up, choose a time to stop. The best time really is when he feels ready. You may be able to help by juggling the outside environment to cut down on stresses such as unwelcome visitors, and by helping arrange distractions so he is enjoyably busy – a holiday may help.
- Because nicotine is so addictive, cutting down does not seem to be that effective. Likewise, changing to lower tar cigarettes is also of little benefit, as evidence suggests that smokers of low tar cigarettes simply inhale more deeply. As a result, some highly dangerous forms of lung cancer actually appear to be higher in smokers of low tar cigarettes.
- Clean up the house, wash clothes and furnishings, and bin all smoking cues, such as ash-trays and lighters.
- Arrange outings so as to avoid places or situations where he usually smokes – visit new places, including non-smoking restaurants.
- Likewise, try and plan social events so you are with people who do not smoke.
- Write out a list of reasons to stop, and write it out again every day along with affirmations or a cassette ('I, *name*, am now a non-smoker').
- Put the money saved to one side and plan a holiday or just spend it on other treats.
- Smoking cessation aids may help. Nicotine replacements such as gum, patches and inhalers are available from your pharmacist, or ask your GP about nicotine replacement therapy, which research suggests can double the chances of giving up. Gum will ease the craving most quickly (good if you are only severely tempted at certain times), while patches provide a steady dose which may be better for the all-day smoker.
- Your GP can also advise on medication. The anti-depressant drug bupropion hydrochloride (trade name Zyban) is now also used to help people stop smoking. Some studies suggest it is more effective than a nicotine patch. It has similar effects on the brain to nicotine, which means there is a small risk of seizure in some people. It can also cause a dry mouth and insomnia and is not recommended for people with eating disorders. Treatment should start at least a week before you stop smoking.

- Encourage him to drink plenty of water throughout the day, and if he gets a sudden craving give him some healthy snacks to chew on such as carrot and celery sticks, grapes and fruit pieces.
- Encourage him to exercise – swimming, jogging, underwater basket-weaving, anything that keeps him busy.
- Believe he can do it. Unconsciously or consciously expecting him to fail can undermine his efforts. Offer loads of encouragement and support, armed with precise information from a support organization like ASH. Point out that the craving only lasts a short while and that the body does soon readjust.
- He may like to try alternative therapies such as acupuncture, hypnotherapy, massage or aromatherapy.
- Research the available support – research shows it really does make a significant difference to the chances of successfully giving up. Encourage him to join a support group or see a smoking cessation counsellor. Your GP should be able to refer you.

Sleep well

Insomnia takes different forms – an inability to go to sleep after going to bed, using pills or alcohol to get to sleep, waking up often during the night, early waking, or waking up unrefreshed. Most people have probably experienced a run of bad nights, for example before starting a new job. Usually what happens is that the body catches up with a period of deeper sleep once the period of tension is over. Insomnia lasting for weeks or months, however, is believed to affect up to 15 per cent of the population, and can be implicated with, or lead to, further mental and physical health problems.

Because of this, it may be worth involving your doctor to help sort out insomnia – do not assume that it is 'all in his mind' if the insomnia drags on and is obviously making him miserable. Insomnia can also be a symptom of depression and anxiety as well as of some medical conditions such as heart disease, breathing problems and high blood pressure. Symptoms such as shortness of breath or pain combined with insomnia should take him straight to his GP. Some prescription drugs such as diuretics and some beta-blockers can cause sleep problems.

Much insomnia relates to 'unfinished business' from the day – feelings that have not been expressed or dealt with, tasks that have not been done – or to more long-term stress, such as an unsatisfactory situation at work. Obviously, sorting out the underlying cause will help the insomnia, although this may involve learning some stress-management or relaxation techniques to help sort out what are, and are not, reasonable expectations.

However, physical factors can make a difference to how well he sleeps, as well as sleep habits. Good sleep hygiene (i.e. healthy sleeping habits) goes a long way to beating insomnia.

How to help

- Going to bed at the same time every night, boring though it sounds, is one of the most important factors in establishing good sleep habits as it helps to regulate your circadian rhythm, the internal biological clock that governs your sleep/wake cycles. Going to bed before midnight makes the most of the deep sleep that occurs early in the night.
- If you do not have one, try and establish a soothing pre-bedtime routine together, such as a light snack, listening to music, or having a chat.
- Vigorous physical exercise in the evening can leave people 'wound up' and unable to sleep, so if he does exercise late in the day, suggest he keeps it mild or does it earlier. An evening walk or swim together is ideal.
- Do not have a large meal late at night. Make your main meal earlier in the day – lunchtime or early evening – and have a milky drink and snack at bedtime such as a banana, or peanut butter sandwich, or a bowl of cereal. All of these contain the amino acid tryptophan which helps your body produce the sleep hormone melatonin.
- Keep the bedroom for relaxation, sleep and sex. Do not store work-related items or papers in a corner. Try not to have discussions about money or moving house there, try and discuss any problems before you go to bed and ideally do not have a TV.
- Check external factors which can affect sleep such as noise, light, heat, cold, discomfort. A new bed may help; one survey showed that even poor sleepers slept better in a new bed than in one that

was ten years old. A bed should support your back while allowing your spine to settle into its natural slight 'S' shape when you lie flat.

- Cigarettes, alcohol, junk food and caffeine can all overstimulate. A late night cigarette can delay sleep by half an hour or more even in heavy smokers. It is worth avoiding coffee after 2 p.m. if it seems to have an effect.
- Relaxation techniques may be worth exploring. One study showed insomniacs who combined meditation with sleep hygiene techniques fell asleep 77 per cent faster than before. Biofeedback, which uses medical monitoring equipment to help you recognize when you are tense, may help you relax if insomnia is due to anxiety or stress.
- Try traditional natural herbal remedies such as valerian, hops and passiflora. Antihistamine-based over-the-counter sleeping pills are also useful, non-addictive, short-term remedies. Melatonin, a hormone which helps regulate the body's circadian rhythm, is available on prescription (in the UK) in synthetic form and acts as a mild natural sleeping pill.
- Your GP can prescribe sleeping pills as a short-term measure if he is desperate (they are addictive and can cause irritability and tiredness so other approaches are worth trying first).
- Do not use alcohol to get to sleep – it cuts down on the amount of REM sleep he has, a vital time in which the brain sorts out problems, and so can leave him unrefreshed and still tired.

Snoring and sleep apnoea

Snoring, when breathing through the mouth makes the tissue at the back of the throat vibrate, affects up to half of all men, and is more likely if he is overweight and unfit, with a shirt-collar size of 17 or more. Drinking and smoking also contribute to snoring. Enlarged tonsils, adenoids or a blocked nose can all cause temporary snoring.

More serious is sleep apnoea, which happens if the airway becomes completely blocked, causing frequent waking, sometimes gasping for breath. Sleep apnoea is potentially dangerous as it carries an increased risk of high blood pressure, stroke and heart attack, so he must see his GP. It also causes daytime sleepiness, as the man wakes up several times a night without always realizing it, morning headaches, moodiness, and poor memory.

How to help him with snoring and sleep apnoea

- Help him pay attention to lifestyle issues as discussed in this chapter. Ideally, he should lose weight and get fit, stop smoking and drinking and avoid sleeping pills, all of which can make snoring and sleep apnoea worse.
- See if he can sleep on his side as he is more likely to snore if he sleeps on his back. Propping him with pillows may help.
- Ask your pharmacist or GP about nasal clips or strips.
- Medical treatments include an air pressure device called the CPAP (continuous positive airway pressure) device which can bring about dramatic improvements in apnoea sufferers.
- Men with severe apnoea can have surgery to cauterize the soft palate but this is usually a last resort.

10

Psychological and emotional health

Psychological and emotional health are dirty words where men are concerned, but responsible for much silent illness. Depression, for example, is widespread but under-recognized among men – an estimated one in five develop clinical depression at some point during their lives. Anxiety and obsessive-compulsive disorders are also surprisingly common. The macho attitude is often what underlies men's reluctance to look after their physical health, too, so emotional health needs to be tackled for optimum well-being.

According to some experts, many men may not realize they are suffering psychologically because they do not display classic symptoms such as exhaustion, panic attacks or bursting into tears. The theory is that psychological problems in men, such as anxiety and depression, may take different forms to problems in women. Men may be more likely to show psychological distress by their behaviour, such as silence and sulking, and especially dangerous behaviour such as aggressive driving, drinking too much, and becoming more argumentative and even violent, maybe towards their families. This does not apply to all men, of course. Emotional literacy and the ability to verbalize feelings varies widely across both sexes.

Taking the emotions-as-behaviour theory further, however, some therapists believe that much behaviour we take for granted as being normally male, such as the odd fisticuffs or, more voguishly, going through a 'mid-life crisis', are in fact symptoms of disturbance imposed by society's expectations of men to be tough and self-reliant. This seems to be particularly true of certain groups, such as those brought up in poverty, or black men.

Getting help, whether it is going to a doctor or taking medication, in their minds, is a sign of weakness – sometimes a killer sign, because as discussed in previous chapters, it often prevents men getting medical help until it is too late. Holding in emotions can have bad effects on health too. Recent studies indicate that people prone to rage are more likely to suffer from heart disease, high blood pressure, and early death.

On the positive side, looking after emotional health leads to greater self-esteem and control, as well as greater health – studies have shown that men who are willing to express their feelings have stronger immune systems and are less susceptible to diseases such as heart disease, asthma and arthritis.

Recognizing and coping with feelings

Recognizing feelings means breaking through a layer of invulnerability and so can be especially difficult for men. The man who finds it difficult to talk about his feelings but sits seething in front of the TV is a laughable stereotype, yet all too alive, as Julie's story shows:

> If he was in a 'bad mood', Scott would come home from work, eat, and plonk down in front of the TV with a face like thunder. This might go on for days or weeks and could happen after a bad day at work, or a row with me. The worst time was when he had to attend some prostate tests at the local hospital – he kept silence for weeks. It was only after a few cans of beer or after we'd shared a bottle of wine for dinner that it would all come out.

Men may block or deny feelings in a number of ways – through embarrassment, shame, anger, or just being numb or not in touch with their emotions. Bottling up anger or not showing emotion openly are classic male attributes or, conversely, exploding with rage after a build-up of negative emotions which he does not have the skills to express before they become overwhelming.

It can also be hard for women to recognize and accept male feelings. Strong emotion in men can be frightening for women, especially if, as often happens, they feel that they are responsible for their partner's happiness and the way he feels.

However, accepting all emotions including the negative is an important part of emotional health rather than ignoring them, denying them or losing them through work or heavy drinking. Anger, for example, is a kind of energy which can be channelled to change the situation that is causing the frustration. Grief and sadness too have their value.

Some women also need to realize that there is often a gap between feelings and their expression. Feelings do not always have to be acted upon – the man who comes home in a towering rage and says he wants to kill his boss is not necessarily going to follow the action through. While acceptance of his feelings certainly does not mean you have to put up with any bullying, his emotions are there for a reason, and it may be helpful to think of them as important messengers from his deeper self to which attention needs to be paid.

Matt had developed a morbid fear of illness over the past 18 months. After several fruitless trips to the doctor's, his partner Julie was becoming impatient and insisted he look at the deeper reasons for his fear. After discussing it with her, Matt realized his hypochondria was due to an unrealized fear of 'dying in harness' in a job he hated. He also had a lot of anger towards his boss. He was able to make plans for changing his employment, which he eventually did.

What you can do

- Just listening can be immensely helpful to the man who wants to talk – and who may often talk himself into a solution with very little help from you. Interrupting, or not attending, are two prime ways of discouraging this process.
- Do not feel it is incumbent on you always to come up with some judgement, or to place or interpret your partner's emotions.
- Likewise, if he wants to talk about 'negative' feelings, you do not necessarily have to keep reassuring him or telling him that everything will be all right.
- See what practical steps you or he can take to change the circumstances behind the feelings – work rage, for example, as in Matt's case described above.

Depression

Depression is common, affecting around one in 20 of people. While traditionally three times as many women as men suffer from depression, rates of depression among men are rising, as those in women decrease, maybe due to social pressures on men to be competitive and successful in the face of increasing male unemployment and the increasing presence of women in the workplace.

Depression can run in families, so that he is up to three times more likely to develop depression if he has a parent or sibling who has or has had depression. Stressful life events such as loss of a job or the arrival of a baby can also trigger depression, as can illness, such as heart disease or cancer. The male tendency to bury feelings in drink rather than talking about problems may also contribute to some depression. Men may suffer various specific types of depression, including manic depression, seasonal affective disorder and post-natal depression.

Depression can have both psychological and physical symptoms, for example:

- problems with memory or concentration
- constantly feeling sad or unhappy – these feelings may be worse at a particular time of day, especially early in the morning
- loss of interest and/or pleasure in life
- feeling worthless and guilty even if rationally he knows it is not justified
- difficulties with memory and concentration
- loss of appetite
- weight loss
- feeling emotionally vulnerable and sensitive, maybe crying
- sleeping difficulties and early waking
- loss of interest in sex
- thoughts of suicide.

Sometimes, instead of recognizing that a man is depressed, partners may think that he has changed, or that he is 'not himself' in ways that are not easy to define. Having a partner who is depressed can be very wearing for you, and for the whole family, as Stacie says:

At first I just thought Tom was 'off' or maybe suffering the effects of a virus. He seemed to have two moods – either very picky and irritable and grumbling at everything; or withdrawn and morose. As the depression went on, the morose mood prevailed and it became difficult to get him to do ordinary things like see friends together or even go for a walk, which previously had been our main weekend relaxation. I was sympathetic at first but as the months went by it really began to get to me to the extent I felt it was ruining my life too.

What you can do

- Get him to see his doctor if he has five or more of the symptoms of depression above, particularly if they have persisted for two weeks or more. Your partner may not realize he is depressed – a common manifestation of depression – but it is all the more important to make him go for help. Because he is depressed, he may feel too worthless or apathetic to seek (or feel he deserves) help.
- Make sure your doctor understands the reason for the visit. Research shows that doctors miss around half of the cases of depression presented to them at the first consultation.
- Try and ensure your partner complies with any medication prescribed. Bear in mind he may have to wait two to six weeks for the effects to be felt.
- Ask the doctor about psychological therapy to explore deeper issues which medication cannot resolve.
- Pay attention to the family diet. Include more fruit and vegetables and complex carbohydrates and try and avoid sugar and refined white flour. Also ensure he gets enough B vitamins, especially folic acid. A deficiency of folic acid has recently been linked to heart disease and Alzheimer's disease, but could also be important in depression. Folic acid is in fortified breakfast cereals and green vegetables, wheatgerm, liver, dark leafy vegetables.
- Try and get him out into sunlight or daylight – some depression is thought to be due to low levels of serotonin in the brain. Sunlight striking the retina boosts the production of serotonin (see 'Further reading'). He should remove any glasses for at least 20 minutes.
- The anti-depressant effect of exercise is well-documented, so get him to do what he can – he may be less able to exercise if he is depressed but a walk with you is good even if he cannot manage to join that gym or meet his friends for football.
- Herbal remedies may be helpful, such as St John's wort (which

108

can cause photosensitivity in sunshine) and 5-hydroxytryptophan (5-HT), the chemical from which serotonin is made in the body. Do not take at the same time as prescribed anti-depressants.

- Bear in mind that depression can recur so try and discuss long-term preventative strategies such as overall lifestyle, medication and therapy.

Mid-life crisis

Does the 'male menopause' exist? Experts are divided. There is no doubt that many men do go through a so-called mid-life crisis (as well as many other life crises). Some believe that social and psychological reasons lie behind this. Men who have worked hard all their lives may suddenly find themselves facing retirement, unsure of their status and identity outside work, and socially isolated – 'the unexamined life is not worth living,' as Socrates said.

Some research has suggested that low testosterone may be behind the male menopause. Symptoms of a drop in testosterone include low libido, lack of energy or strength, mood swings such as sadness or irritability, depression, being less effective at work, or frequent drowsiness after the evening meal (symptoms which may mimic those of clinical depression).

Research at the Medical Research Council's Human Reproductive Sciences Unit in Edinburgh suggests that drops in testosterone may cause male mood swings at any age – the so-called 'irritable male syndrome', with grumpiness and irritability, low sex drive and social withdrawal. It is believed that stress such as bereavement, divorce or illness may cause these falling testosterone levels – animal studies show that testosterone levels fall when stress increases the levels of the hormone corticosteroid.

Before he rushes off to the doctor for some extra testosterone, medical experts have not yet agreed on this theory. Some experts say changes in testosterone levels in men are far smaller than the dramatic swings seen in some of the animals studied, for example, rams. While there is growing awareness of the effect of testosterone on men, it is not as well studied as the impact of hormones on women. Testosterone replacement therapy (TRT) itself is as controversial as the idea of a male menopause – some men swear by it and say it has given them a wonderful boost in vitality and well-being, but worries about side effects include testosterone's links with prostate cancer. And medical experts fear that extra testosterone may not cause, but might stimulate, the growth of any prostate cancer that already exists.

If he is over 40 and is suffering symptoms as described above, he could consult his doctor about TRT or anti-depressants. It may also help to focus on life issues such as unfulfilled goals and long-term ambitions, either with you or with a trained counsellor (see 'Types of therapy', below).

Getting help for yourself

There may come a time when you feel you are running out of resources and patience, and that you can no longer bear the full weight of your partner's emotions alone. Maybe you feel you are going round in circles, or that you are not getting through, or that the situation has become too serious for you to manage. Do not underestimate the amount of emotional energy it can take to support someone who is constantly depressed, or who has other psychological problems. This is particularly important if any mental disturbance in your partner takes the form of domestic violence.

It is important that you get help – and, above all, that you do not become socially isolated as a result of any problems or manipulation on your partner's part. Hang on to your friends, and stay involved in your usual activities. Do not always anxiously rush back home to check that he is all right.

If you need help, your GP remains a good starting point and may be able to advise you on specific available support, or may prescribe medication as a short-term coping measure. Your GP can also refer you to a counsellor or psychotherapist. See 'Useful addresses' for other groups which may be helpful.

Helping him get the best out of his doctor

As already stated in this book, men are not great at going to the doctor. Men aged 16–24 have a health check every seven years, while men between 25 and 39 have one every five years. Fear, embarrassment and macho attitudes keep too many men away until it is too late.

It may save time and trouble if you help him prepare for visits. First, decide clearly on why he is going. This may sound obvious, but sometimes there may be two or three issues which he may want to discuss. Write down any separate health issues in a list along with specific symptoms – some men may need help on this as men tend to have a poorer vocabulary for describing symptoms than do women. Also write down any questions.

You may or may not want to accompany him, depending on what you both feel. Either way, he can let his doctor know at the beginning of the appointment that he has two or three issues he needs to discuss.

One idea is to have a small notebook or diary you keep specifically for noting health symptoms and doctor's visits. Use it to write down what the doctor says, too. Here are some other tips:

- Speak plainly – while many doctors are highly intuitive, they are not mind readers.
- Make sure you both understand what your doctor says and, if not, ask questions until you do.
- Do not always expect an instant diagnosis. Tests and investigation can take time.

Types of therapy

The advent of life coaching or consulting has challenged perceptions of therapy as being for the birds. While some men respond well to more 'traditional' long-term therapy, lying on a couch for an hour a week is seen as old-fashioned and ineffective by many. Life coaching – a series of talks with a trained person who helps you to achieve specific goals and change specific situations in your life – may work better for men (and businesses) who want results. This emphasis on goal-orientated therapy can work for people who know what is unsatisfactory in their lives and are willing to take action to change it.

Group therapy may also work well for some men, and is often recommended for men to help them counteract the feelings of isolation that tend to be present as a particular feature of male health.

Behavioural therapies may be helpful in dealing with problems on a deeper level. As men may express distress by their behaviour, rather than simply a change of mood, behavioural therapies may help deal with problems on two levels – the surface problem such as drinking too much or compulsive working; and any underlying depression, anxiety, or other issues. Cognitive behavioural therapy, especially effective for depression, looks at thinking habits or patterns which may underlie depression, and works at changing them. It can be effective for other negative behaviours such as compulsive eating, drinking or gambling, phobias or sexual problems. Ask your GP or look for private counsellors. Obviously, as with all therapy, he does need to be motivated and want to change.

Human potential therapies such as art therapy, existential, gestalt and primal therapies and transactional analysis focus on personal development rather than on treating symptoms. Like life coaching, this type of therapy may help a person decide what he wants to do, and support him in achieving it.

It is worth looking round before deciding on a therapist or group. It is important he feels comfortable with whoever he has chosen, and that he is not taken in by any heavy sell, blackmailing or being made to feel guilty. A man who is looking for therapy is likely to be at a vulnerable point in his life, and the last thing he needs from therapy is more psychological suffering from a therapist or group who have a heavy-duty moral agenda. Remember you will get the fall-out! Groups and therapists come in many different shapes and sizes, so if he does not feel happy, he should move on.

He can also go privately (see 'Useful addresses' for counselling organizations that can help you find a therapist). Although expensive, this does give a wider range of choice, with the risk that he ends up seeing someone who is insufficiently qualified and may end up doing more harm than good. A chat on the phone, or an initial five-minute meeting, is a good idea before he commits himself.

Counselling may not be for everyone. Simon checked out Relate and a couple of private therapists before deciding against it.

My initial dislike of counselling wasn't that I was afraid of talking about my feelings; I just felt that it was a shame that the only way I could get anyone to listen to me was to pay them. I didn't like Relate because the therapist was quite insistent that I bring my partner along if the therapy was to be effective and while fundamentally we do have a good relationship, I wanted my own space at that point. I talked to two other therapists three times each. They were lovely people, but I didn't like the artificiality of the setting – paying for empathy. I felt I ought to be able to manage with my own resources and friends. In the end I decided I wanted to get to know people in a more equal or normal social setting. My next door neighbour was a keen archer and always inviting me along to give it a try. I didn't stay with it but I did check out a few other local clubs and just taking that action seemed to be the turning point in the way I felt and how I handled my life. For a while I tried out a few things, then we decided to move to another part of the country where we felt we would have more in common with the people, and it worked – we've never looked back.

Suicide

Men are about three times more likely to kill themselves than women, according to official figures from the Office for National Statistics, and suicide is now the second cause of death in young men and the fourth leading cause of death – since 1981, the suicide rate has increased by 55 per cent among young men aged 15–24. It is believed that the male tendency not to express feelings, and to drink as a way of dealing with emotions, are factors in this. Divorced men are more likely than any other group to kill themselves, with social isolation being a major factor.

Suicide needs to be taken seriously as a risk in depression. Sadly, men often ensure that the deed is carried out irrevocably, for example, by means of firearms, rather than being a 'cry for help', for example with overdose as in women.

Do not ignore any warning signs in your partner, such as severe depression or talk of suicide. Consult your doctor or call a helpline such as SANELINE or the Samaritans (see 'Useful addresses').

Living through bereavement and other grief

Bereavement can take many forms but nearly always involves some shift in identity and vulnerability. People or situations which were perhaps taken for granted suddenly go or change, and the whole viewpoint of life has to be redefined, a process which can take months or years.

Malcom, 42, lost his father in January and in April was diagnosed with Crohn's disease. Although his condition was not life-threatening, it was severe enough, and he felt he needed to grieve both for his father and for his own lost past, including the time when he had been healthy. Losing his father and his health were both bereavements, bringing home his mortality in a way which had never happened before.

A partner can be an enormous support during a time of grief, so long as she or he does not try to be everything to the one who is grieving, or trivialize the loss. Grief must run its course and no one, however supportive, can take it away – indeed, some people cherish their grief as a precious link to the person or situation that was lost.

Being happy

While happiness may not be on the prescription your GP hands you, it is a vital ingredient for health. This does not mean mindlessly obeying the classic American farewell – strangely put as a command – of 'Enjoy!' However, a decision to be happy as far as possible has been shown to boost health, while the benefits of positive emotions to health are well-documented.

A vital part of this is a sense of humour, which helps build psychological resistance in an age when people are increasingly pushed to the edge of their resources by the demands of everyday modern life. Humour, traditionally suppressed by modern society under pressures to 'be serious' or 'stop fooling around', has been shown to boost immunity by speeding up the creation of new immune cells and the production of 'T' lymphocytes and gamma interferon. It lowers levels of the stress hormone cortisol and contributes to muscle relaxation, pain management, lower blood pressure, improved circulation and respiratory function and less inflammation and infection. Laughing clubs exist in several countries round the world, including India, while American hospitals now have a humour room or trolley which is wheeled from ward to ward by volunteers.

While attempts to manufacture humour may seem a bit self-conscious, they do act as valuable reminders to see the funny side of life from time to time. Play, or playfulness, is central to sound emotional health.

Friends

Experts agree that healthy men need a network of family and friends, and that lack of contact with others is a common source of trouble. This may not mean a quick drink with tennis partners, or work social events. Men need like-minded souls with whom they can speak freely, and who will really listen and respond.

Simon, mentioned above, found he was quite socially isolated, and that most people seemed too busy to give him the time of day. He was also quite selective in who he wanted to mix with. Finding soul mates was not easy!

When I talked to other men, I always felt constricted to keep anything I shared male, whether rightly or wrongly. Talking about feelings or showing vulnerability was definitely not on. I found these constraints boring.

To find the type of people I could feel at ease with, I had to be quite creative and adventurous and do things I wouldn't normally do. In the past, I would just wait and let people drift into my life. This time I really explored the local society quite thoroughly. I decided I would try and go to things just once to see if I liked them, like the film society – that was an unexpected success as I met a couple of people there I felt at ease with. I also did some supply teaching and found a few people tucked away in educational establishments round the place – the reason I hadn't met them before was that they were at work. Apart from anything else, this really took the pressure off my partner Maggie to be my best and only friend.

His last remark highlights a common problem – being 'taken hostage' by the man against the world. You may be able to help your man expand his social circle by taking the social initiative and ensuring that people are regularly invited to the house. Events like these provide a good chance for your partner to sound out people he likes to see if they might be candidates for friendship, and to gauge how they react if he talks about subjects he enjoys.

Another idea is to make contact with old friends from previous jobs or from college or school. Remind him that while it may take courage to take the first step, he may find that other men need support and friendship just as he does.

Conclusion

Men's health is a huge topic. It is hoped that this book has provided an introduction to the subject which will draw attention to some of its main areas, particularly lifestyle issues and preventative care. As already stressed, these are the areas where men today need to sit up and pay attention, and to fight against a culture which invites them to an early grave.

The time has definitely come for men to take responsibility for their health into their own hands, not to rely on women, or on a last-hope dash to the doctor to patch up a lifetime of poor life habits. Hopefully this book will have given you a few suggestions on how to help your man to start looking after himself, and how to improve in areas where he is already taking action.

If you do want to explore the subject further, several good resources have sprung up since alarm bells about male health started sounding a few years ago. Other books may look at the subject in more detail or may focus on individual conditions such as prostate disease. Online resources abound, too – in the UK, one of the most comprehensive is www.malehealth.co.uk, which explores several topics in detail, looking at symptoms, causes, treatment and self-help suggestions, while the UK male health policy site is also authoritative (www.menshealthforum.co.uk). Or it may be a case of contacting a support group or an organization for information about a specific problem. Reading suggestions and contact details are given over the next few pages.

Whichever way you go, there is plenty that can be done to brighten the prospects for male health – your future prospects, too, in terms of having a healthy, energetic companion in later years. In 1920, the lifespan gender gap was just one year, in contrast to today's 7- to 14-year gap. This shows that men are not necessarily inherently weaker than women – just that their living skills have gone wrong somewhere. Spending too much time indoors and sedentary, eating too much of the wrong foods, drinking and smoking too much – they are all familiar, and all capable of being

117

tackled. Some men are tackling them. Figures suggesting that the gap is on the wane perhaps reflect men's growing awareness of their health needs today. If everyone took some action in these areas alone, we might see the lifespan gap shrink back to one of complete sexual equality.

Useful addresses

Acne Support Group
Web site: www.m2w3.com/acne/home.html
PO Box 230
Hayes
Middlesex UB4 0UT
Tel: 020 8561 6868

Alcohol Concern
Web site: www.alcoholconcern.org.uk
Waterbridge House
32–36 Loman Street
London SE1 0EE
Tel: 020 7928 7377
Email: contact@alcoholconcern.org.uk

Alcoholics Anonymous
Web site: www.alcoholics-anonymous.org.uk
PO Box 1
Stonebow House
Stonebow
York YO1 7NJ
Tel: 0845 769 7555

ASH (Action on Smoking and Health)
Web site: www.ash.org.uk
102 Clifton Street
London EC2A 4HW
Tel: 020 7739 5902
Email: action.smoking.health@dial.pipex.com

British Heart Foundation
Web site: www.bhf.org.uk
14 Fitzhardinge Street
London W1H 6DH
Tel: 020 7935 0185

British Nutrition Foundation
Web site: www.nutrition.org.uk
High Holborn House
52–54 High Holborn
London WC1V 6RQ
Tel: 020 7404 6504
Email: postbox@nutrition.org.uk

British Snoring and Sleep Apnoea Association
Web site: www.britishsnoring.co.uk
1 Duncroft Close
Reigate
Surrey RH2 9DE
Tel: 01737 245638
Email: info@britishsnoring.co.uk

CancerBACUP
Web site: www.cancerbacup.org.uk
3 Bath Place
Rivington Street
London EC2A 3JR
Tel: 020 7696 9003

Depression Alliance
Web site: www.depressionalliance.org
35 Westminster Bridge Rd
London SE1 7JB
Tel: 020 7633 0557

Diabetes UK
Web site: www.diabetes.org.uk
10 Parkway
London NW1 7AA
Tel: 020 7424 1000
Email: info@diabetes.org.uk

Digestive Disorders Foundation
Web site: www.digestivedisorders.org.uk
3 St Andrews Place
Regents Park
London NW1 4LB
Tel: 020 7486 0341
Email: ddf@digestivedisorders.org.uk

Domestic Violence Intervention Project
Web site: www.dvip.org
PO Box 2838
London W6 9ZE
Tel: 020 8563 7983
Email: info@dvip.org

Drinkline
Tel: 0800 917 8282

Eating Disorders Association
Web site: www.edauk.com
103 Prince of Wales Road
Norwich NR1 1DW
Tel: 0870 770 3256
Adult helpline: 0845 634 1414
Youthline: 0845 634 7650
Email: info@edauk.com

www.embarrassingproblems.co.uk
(embarrassing problems such as bad breath)

emental-health
www.emental-health.com
(mental health)

FMS Healthcare
PO Box 6940
Nottingham NG2 7XP

Impotence Association
Web site: www.impotence.org.uk
PO Box 10296
London SW17 9WH
Tel: 020 8767 7791
Email: theia@btinternet.com

International Stress Management Association
Web site: www.isma.org.uk
PO Box 348
Waltham Cross EN8 8ZL
Tel: 07000 780430
Email: stress@isma.org.uk

ISSUE: The National Fertility Association
Web site: www.issue.co.uk
114 Lichfield Street
Walsall
West Midlands WS1 1SZ
Tel: 01922 722888
Email: webmaster@issue.co.uk

National Eczema Society
Web site: www.eczema.org
Hill House
Highgate Hill
London N19 5NA
Tel: 020 7281 3553
Helpline: 0870 241 3604 (Mon–Fri 1–4 p.m.)

NHS Direct
Web site: www.nhsdirect.nhs.uk
Tel: 0845 4647
(online information and 24-hour telephone helpline run by nurses
trained to give advice over the phone)

Orchid Cancer Appeal
Web site: www.orchid-cancer.org.uk
(for men with prostate or testicular cancer)

Prostate Cancer Charity
Web site: www.prostate-cancer.org.uk
3 Angel Walk
Hammersmith
London W6 9HX
Tel: 0845 300 8383

Prostate Help Association
Web site: www.pha.u-net.com
PHA(W)
Langworth
Lincoln LN3 5DF

Prostate Research Campaign UK
Web site: www.prostate-research.org.uk
36 The Drive
Northwood
Middlesex HA6 1HP
Email: info@prostate-research.org.uk

Quitline
Tel: 0800 002200
(for advice and information on stopping smoking)

Quitsmokinguk.com
Web site: www.quitsmokinguk.com
Email: feedback@quitsmokinguk.com

Relate
Web site: www.relate.org.uk
Herbert Gray College
Little Church Street
Rugby
Warwickshire CV21 3AP
Tel: 01788 573241
Email: enquiries@national.relate.org.uk

The Samaritans
Web site: www.samaritans.org
Tel: 08457 909090
Email: jo@samaritans.org

SANELINE
Tel: 0345 678 000

SimplyFood
Web site: www.simplyfood.com
(for food, nutrition and healthy eating information)

Slimming World
Web site: www.slimming-world.co.uk
Tel: 0870 330 7733
Email: info@slimming-world.co.uk

The Stroke Association
Web site: www.stroke.org.uk
Stroke House
Whitecross Street
London EC1Y 8JJ
Helpline: 0845 30 33 100
Email: info@stroke.org.uk

Web sites – UK

www.malehealth.co.uk – information about male health

www.menshealthforum.co.uk – UK male health policy site for male health

www.jr2ox.ac.uk/bandolier – Bandolier, an internet journal covering men's health

www.mensproject.org/malelink.html – The Male Link

www.menshealthnetwork.org

www.menshealthnews.com

www.rationalrecovery.net

www.interconnections.co.uk – Interconnections – holistic living and complementary therapies

www.dipex.org – DIPEx (Database of Individual Patient Experience)

America

Men's Health Network
PO Box 75972
Washington DC 20013
Phone: 202-543-MHN1 (6461)
www.menshealthnetwork.org

Web sites – America

Men's Health
http://www.plainsense.com/Health/Mens/

Male Health Center
www.malehealthcenter.com

Men Web
www.vix.cim/menmag/mensheal.htm
Articles on various health topics

Impotence Resource Site
www.impotence.org/

The National Men's Resource
www.menstuff.org
An international resource on more than 100 men's issues

Prostate Health
www.prostatehealth.com

Testicular Cancer Resource Center
www.inform.acor.org/disease/tc/
http://rex.nci.nih.gov/WTNK_PUBS/testicular/index.htm

Further reading

Apple, Michael and Rowena Gaunt, *Men's Health Handbook*, Metro Books, London 1998

Armstrong, Joe, *Men's Health: The Commonsense Approach*, Gill and Macmillan Newleaf, Dublin 1999

Baker, Peter, *The Optimum Health Guide For Men*, Mitchell Beazley, London 2001

Banks, Ian, *Ask Dr Ian About Men's Health*, The Blackstaff Press, Belfast 1997

Beare, Helen and Neil Priddy, *The Cancer Guide for Men*, Sheldon Press 1999

Bradford, Nikki, *Men's Health Matters: The Complete A–Z of Male Health*, Vermilion, London 1995

Brewer, Sarah, *The Complete Book of Men's Health*, Thorsons, London 1997, reprint 1999

Carroll, Steve, *The Which? Guide to Men's Health*, Which? Books 1994, third edition 1999

Forem, Jack, *et al.*, *The Complete Book of Men's Health*, Mitchell Beazley, London 1999

Hopcroft, Keith and Alistair Moulds, *A Bloke's Diagnose It Yourself Guide to Health*, Oxford University Press, Oxford 2000

Lazarides, Linda, *The Waterfall Diet*, Piatkus Books, London, reprint 2000

Phillips, Katharine A., *The Broken Mirror: Understanding and Treating Body Dysmorphic Disorder*, Oxford University Press, Oxford 1996

Pollack, William, *Real Boys: Rescuing Our Sons from the Myths of Boyhood*, Owl Books 1999

Pollard, Jim, *All Right, Mate? An Easy Intro to Men's Health*, Vista, London 1999

Pope, Harrison G., *et al.*, *The Adonis Complex: The Secret Crisis of Male Body Obsession*, The Free Press 2000

Rodwell, Lee, *You and Your Prostate*, Self-Help Direct Publishing 1997

FURTHER READING

Savill, Jonathan and Richard Smedley, *No More Mr Fat Guy: The Nutrition and Fitness Programme for Men!*, Vermilion, London 1999

Smith, Alex, *Essentials for Men: Health and Fitness*, Mitchell Beazley, London 2000

Smith, Tom, *Coping Successfully with Prostate Cancer*, Sheldon Press, London 2002

Index